Ethical Issues in Nursing and Midwifery Practice

Also by Win Tadd and published by Macmillan

Chadwick, R and Tadd, W (1992) *Ethics and Nursing Practice: A Case Study Approach*

Ethical Issues in Nursing and Midwifery Practice

Perspectives from Europe

Edited by

Win Tadd

MACMILLAN

First published 1998 by
MACMILLAN PRESS LTD
Houndmills, Basingstoke, Hampshire RG21 6XS
and London
Companies and representatives
throughout the world

ISBN 0–333–71005–3 paperback

A catalogue record for this book is available from the British Library.

This book is printed on paper suitable for recycling and made from fully managed and sustained forest sources.

10 9 8 7 6 5 4 3 2 1
07 06 05 04 03 02 01 00 99 98

Editing and origination by
Aardvark Editorial, Mendham, Suffolk

Printed in Malaysia

For Vic, Beccy and Andrew,
my inspiration

Contents

Foreword

I must admit I find the idea of ethics daunting and I am sure I am not the only one. It sounds such a dry, philosophical topic, providing scholars, priests and hermits with ample opportunity for learned speculation but bearing little relationship to the real world – particularly the messy, chaotic world of health care, which to its practitioners seems more real than most. Win Tadd and the contributors she has brought together in this book clearly disagree, and perhaps they share my view that just as politics is too important to be left to politicians and medicine too important to be left to doctors, so ethics is too important to be left to ethicists.

The recent growth in health professionals' interest in ethics has been striking, and has gradually widened to include nurses and others at all levels and in all areas of practice, the target audience for this book. Far from being consigned to a dusty, unwanted corner of the curriculum, ethical issues are increasingly prominent in everyday discussions about health care. The reasons are many and varied, but undoubtedly include the changing role and greater autonomy of nurses, who can no longer hide behind others' authority but are, as their regulatory body points out, individually accountable to the public for maintaining safe standards of care. At the same time, rising demands and inadequate health care resources often force practitioners and managers into making priority choices which they find difficult or even unacceptable.

The ethical issues are unavoidable – part of the fabric of human life. In health care they arise at policy level, with governments deciding which services, professions or research should receive most funding, or devolving those tricky rationing decisions to local level. One topical example is assisted conception: should this be provided by the National Health Service or should couples go private? Is it acceptable that availability of the state-funded service should depend on your postcode?

Even more pressing for the practitioner are the ethical issues which constantly arise in their daily work. At every turn they are required to make snap decisions about what to do for whom and how to do it. When staffing levels are low and clients' needs seem endless, how can they choose between competing, sometimes conflicting, demands? Who gets my attention first, the woman screaming in the corner or the one next to her in a wet bed? What do I say when the patient has not been given information about his diagnosis but the family has? These are real dilemmas which the practitioner often feels obliged to solve (or sidestep) in isolation, at the risk of being chided or punished for making the 'wrong' choice.

Any book which aims to stimulate debate on ethics in nursing is therefore to be welcomed. This one has a particularly innovative emphasis on the transcultural dimension. By taking a European perspective, with authors, case studies and examples from a wide range of countries, it enables us to flush out our taken-for-granted views and examine them in the light of others' experiences. It reminds us of the diversity of ethical views within our own multicultural, multi-ethnic societies: no homogeneous societies now exist, if indeed they ever did.

Comfortingly, though, there may be as much that unites us as divides us. As Tadd points out, 'transcultural ethics relies on a moral sense which originates from our shared humanity and shared human experiences... these elements of humanity all arise from basic fears, beliefs and values which are common across all cultures'. I found this to be true in my last job at the World Health Organization, where as Regional Adviser for Nursing and Midwifery in Europe, I worked with nurses from, and visited them in, many countries – from France and Spain in the west to Russia and Kazakstan in the east, all under the WHO umbrella of 'Europe'.

I observed a multitude of customs, assumptions, nuances, behaviours and attitudes, yet all of us were indeed united by shared humanity and shared experiences – and we also shared a passionate belief in the potential of nursing to cross the divides of gender, race, age, sexuality and so on, to join hands in empathy to alleviate suffering and help each other through hard times. This book provides stimulating, thoughtful and well-informed debate to help us find our way through the moral mazes and thereby enrich our own, our colleagues' and our patients' lives.

JANE SALVAGE, RGN, BA, MSc HonLLD
Editor-in-Chief, *Nursing Times*

Acknowledgements

I owe a debt of gratitude to many people without whose help and support this book would not have been possible. I would first like to thank the contributors who, by their punctuality and diligence, made my task all the easier. Thank you.

Second, I shall be forever grateful to the numerous nurses in the UK and Europe who have shared their thoughts and experiences with me during my many years of teaching. The pleasure has been mine and I am quite certain that I have learnt a lot from them.

Particular thanks go to Richenda Milton-Thompson at Macmillan for her advice, understanding and endless patience in the preparation of this volume and to an anonymous reviewer for a helpful and encouraging critique.

To Marianne Arndt of the University of Stirling and Humboldt University in Germany, thank you for your patient reading of the manuscript and your constructive comments which were enormously helpful.

Finally, I would like to thank members of my family. My parents for their influence and example; my husband Vic, for his patient reading, helpful comments and culinary skills; and my children, Rebecca and Andrew, for just being themselves.

Publisher's acknowledgements

The editor and publishers wish to thank Academic Press: California, for their kind permission to reprint with minor editing, copyright material on pages 23–32 in this volume, from Tadd, W. (1997) 'Nurses' ethics', in Chadwick, R. (ed. in chief), *Encyclopaedia of Applied Ethics*.

About the Contributors

Gosia Brykczynska BA, BSc, RN, RSCN, Cert Ed, RNT, Dip PH, is Lecturer in Philosophy and Ethics at the RCN Institute, London. As a humanities graduate, she specialized in Soviet and East European studies. After working with leprosy patients for the US Public Health Service, she obtained a degree in Nursing Studies from Columbia University in New York City. She is currently undertaking doctoral studies in Philosophy at Heythrop College, London University.

Christine Chilton MA (ed.) BSc, Dip Soc Res, RGN, is a free-lance writer now living in France. After graduating in biochemistry and pharmacology at the University of Sydney, she worked in the Australian pharmaceutical industry before qualifying as a Registered Nurse in Oxford. She also has a postgraduate diploma in social research and a master's degree in health education. Her professional interests include social pharmacology and empowerment through support networks. She is a member of the Editorial Advisory Board of the *Journal of Substance Misuse*.

Helen Crafter MSc, RGN, RM, RMT, is Senior Lecturer/Practitioner in Midwifery at Thames Valley University, London. She has clinical links at Queen Charlotte's and Chelsea Hospitals and in the community in west London. She qualified as a midwife teacher at the University of Surrey/Royal College of Midwives, London. In 1991 she completed an MSc in Health Education at King's College, London and is the author of *Health Promotion in Midwifery* published in 1997.

Kevin Gournay MPhil, PhD, C.Psychol, AFBPsS, RN, is Professor of Mental Health Nursing at the Institute of Psychiatry in London. He is responsible for the London Thorn Nurse Initiative and his clinical work involves him with patients suffering from post-traumatic stress disorder and schizophrenia. He has been a member of many advisory bodies including the current Mental Health Initiative and the Research Advisory Group for the High Security Commissioning Body. He has studied services in Europe, the USA and Australia. He is author of numerous journal articles, book chapters, and books.

Kevin Kendrick MSc, BA(Hons), Dip Soc Admin, Cert Ethics & Theol, Cert Ed, FETC, RGN, EN(G), OTN, is Lecturer in Nursing and Ethics, School of Healthcare Studies, University of Leeds and is a member of the Royal College of Nursing's Ethics Committee. He is currently engaged in research critically exploring the moral dimensions of 'Living Wills' for Age Concern (UK) and is Network Editor for the international journal, *Health Care in Later Life*. He has published widely on the subject of nursing ethics.

Astrid Norberg RN, BA, MA, PhD, is Professor and Head of the Department of Advanced Nursing, Umeå University, Umeå, Sweden. Her research interests mainly concern ethics in nursing care and communication with people with severe dementia. She is a member of the scientific council of the Swedish National Board of Health and Welfare. In 1989 she received the Sofiahemmet prize and the Swedish King's medal, 8th degree (Serafimer), for her contribution to the development of nursing research in Sweden.

Ruth Northway MSc(Econ), RNMH, ENB(805), CertEd(FE), is Lecturer in Nursing Studies at the University of Wales College of Medicine, Cardiff. Prior to entering nurse education she worked as a Clinical Nurse Specialist for people with learning difficulties. She is currently studying for a doctoral degree and her research focuses on discrimination and people with learning difficulties. Both this research and previous studies have included a European dimension.

Jan Reed PhD, RN, is Professor in the Faculty of Health, Social Work and Education at the University of Northumbria, Newcastle. She qualified as a nurse in 1982, after completing a nursing degree at Newcastle Polytechnic, and in 1983 she was appointed as a research nurse in a care of the elderly unit in Newcastle. Her PhD, completed in 1989, explored how the expectations of older people shaped nurses' assessments of them. Her current research focuses on the care of older people, and she is founding editor of the journal, *Health Care in Later Life*.

Cathy Rowan MA, RM, Adv Dip M, RGN PGCEA, is Senior Lecturer in Midwifery at Thames Valley University, near Slough. She has clinical links at the Royal Berkshire Hospital in Reading and in the community. She is also a Supervisor of Midwives. She worked as a midwife in Africa and India, returning to the UK in 1986. Her MA studies were in medical ethics and her practice interests include issues surrounding pre-natal screening and diagnosis and birth.

June Smail BA(Hons), RGN, RM, DN, CertEd, is Senior Nurse for Primary Care with Gwent Health Authority. Her role involves advising and supporting practice nurses in Gwent on professional, clinical and educational issues, as well as commissioning for primary care and promoting teamwork and multidisciplinary learning in the community. She has many years' experience in community and practice nursing and in developing, and teaching on, Welsh National Board courses. She is an elected member of the UKCC.

Win Tadd PhD, BEd(Hons), RGN, RM, DN (Lond), RCNT, RNT, CertEd (FE), ONC, is an independent Consultant in Health Care Ethics and Education and lectures in the UK and Europe. Her doctoral thesis explored moral agency and the nurse's role and her many publications include *Ethics and Nursing Practice* of which she is co-author. She is an External Post-Doctoral Research Fellow at the Centre for Applied Ethics, University of Wales, Cardiff and with a research scholarship from the UKCC, is currently exploring how nurses use and interpret the Code of Professional Conduct in their practice. She is also a member of a European Union research team examining the relevance of virtue ethics to patients with chronic illness.

Rosie Tope PhD, MEd, RCNT, Cert Ed(FE), DN(Lond), is an independent Consultant in Interdisciplinary Learning and an

External Fellow of the University of Glamorgan. She has a wide experience of teaching nurses as well as other health and social care professions. Her doctoral thesis examined the feasibility of interprofessional learning to enhance collaboration in patient care. She has facilitated a number of interprofessional workshops in the UK and Europe, is a member of various international organizations associated with health care and is author of a number of health service publications.

Verena Tschudin MA, BSc(Hons), RGN, RM, Dip Couns, is Senior Lecturer at the University of East London. She was born in Switzerland but did her nurse training in London after which she worked for many years in oncology in both the UK and Israel. In recent years, with two degrees in ethics, this has become her main area of concern. She has published widely in the fields of counselling and ethics and is editor of the international journal *Nursing Ethics*.

1

Setting the Scene

Win Tadd

Introduction

One of the first questions posed to me when discussing the initial idea for this book was 'Is there a European perspective to nursing ethics or indeed, can there be?' Europe after all is enormous in geographical terms, comprising some 50 or so countries and encompassing a vast diversity of values, languages, cultures, races and religions. At a superficial level therefore, one might be led into thinking that the multicultural, multi-lingual and multi-ethnic continent of Europe is distinguished by its diversity, rather than its similarity. This, of course, is the stuff of ethical relativism which has a long tradition in philo-sophical literature. In simple terms it refers to the notion that moral values are relative to a particular culture and therefore they cannot be judged by the standards of other cultures or societies. In support of such a stance, an ethical relativist might argue that such a position encourages tolerance and humility, as the moral actions of a particular society should only be judged against its own standards and as we can never fully under-stand another culture, then will we ever able to judge it? By pointing to the fact that there is little agreement on what are fundamental moral values, the relativist might also claim that there is no credible alternative to his position.

Such arguments can, however, be challenged on a number of points. For instance, what is a culture? Do cultures approx-imate with geographical or national boundaries? If they do, then why do we hear of the north–south divide in our own country? How was civil war possible in the former Yugoslavia?

Second, is it only from our culture that we acquire moral values or do these arise as a result of religious following, education, family socialization and such like? If so, then one can see that relativism soon disintegrates into ethical subjectivism.

To argue against moral relativism is not simply to argue for moral absolutism which claims that there is only one, true moral code and that anyone who does not accept this is wrong. There is a middle ground provided by moral pluralism which asserts that there may be different moral theories and values which may each apprehend part of the truth of a moral life although none of them has the entire answer. It is through this stance that the possibility of transcultural ethics (Campbell *et al.*, 1997, p. 40) emerges.

Transcultural ethics relies on a moral sense which originates from our shared humanity and shared human experiences, so that although various cultures may express miscellaneous aspects differently, perhaps because of different histories, these elements of humanity all arise from basic fears, beliefs and values which are common across all cultures (Wilson, 1993). Examples of commonly held moral values, include, for example, the view that it is always wrong to take an innocent life and that incest is wrong. The basis for this book, therefore, is that as humans we have more in common than we have dividing us and that by gaining knowledge, understanding and insights into our differences, not only can we learn to respect and value those differences, but we can also learn from them, increasing our own moral repertoire by highlighting our own moral blind spots. Perhaps more importantly, we can learn to live in a moral community where everyone, regardless of culture, race, nationality, religion or gender, is afforded dignity and mutual respect. Thus although there may not be one single European perspective on the ethical issues confronting nurses within their practice, there are many shared values, such as compassion, respect and concern for the weak and vulnerable, among nurses in relation to their practice. There are also common difficulties within the nursing role. Although the nursing role is central to all European health systems, its centrality is rarely acknowledged. As Colliere (1986) identified, many elements of nurses' work, although essential to service users, remain invisible and are therefore disregarded by, for example, studies of nursing workload. In part this is due to the gendered nature of nursing and the classification of nursing as women's work. As such, nurses are invariably excluded from the political and economic decision-making about health care, despite the fact that it is nurses (and patients) who are usually the first to encounter the grim realities which result. As Chilton demonstrates in Chapter 4, even when nurses paticipate in policy decisions they lack the authority and power invested in other professional groups to ensure that their voices are heard or listened to. As tensions increase in European health services due to increased demands, rising costs and reduced resources, the ethical challenges facing nurses will escalate and the need for increased understanding and unity will grow.

Nursing in Europe

The sentiments and views expressed above are of particular importance to European nurses, of whom there are approximately 1,700,000 registered within the countries of the European Union alone (Evers, 1997, p. 172). The pace of change in Europe over recent years has been considerable. The collapse of totalitarian regimes in Eastern and Central Europe, the conflicts and civil unrest in Albania, Northern Ireland and the former Yugoslavia, the redrawing of national and political boundaries, the economic recessions experienced in many European countries, the enlargement of the European Union – none of these events takes place in a vacuum and all of them affect health care and nurses, both individually and as a professional group, in a variety of ways. Also nurses, like everyone else, are members of society and as such are influenced by changes in their environments.

Much of the human pain and destruction caused by armed conflict is witnessed by nurses and health care personnel who try to maintain a service in conditions which most of us cannot begin to imagine. The collapse of political structures means that health services must be rebuilt, invariably in the face of material, technological and human shortages. Old reference points are lost at such times, resulting in uncertainty and the need to renegotiate relationships and rethink philosophies. Most countries in Western Europe are struggling to maintain levels of service, in times of economic recession added to by falling revenue from increasingly ageing societies and the escalating costs of technologically advanced treatments for which the public expectation is rising. The move to market-based economies, regardless of where this is happening, inevitably results in winners and losers in the health stakes. Resources, when available, are prioritized and frequently it is the most vulnerable, the elderly, the chronically ill, the poor as well as children and women whose needs are unmet. Diseases thought to be long eradicated, like tuberculosis and malnutrition, have begun to re-emerge even in the wealthier countries of Europe. Worsening violence in our societies both as a result of crime and civil wars results not only in physical injury but psychological trauma. Illnesses and health needs whose existence was denied by totalitarian regimes, such as the AIDS epidemic and the plight of people with learning disabilities (mental handicap) in Romania, are now evident and must be dealt with. Across Europe, it is the millions of nurses who have to face these challenges and difficulties on a daily basis. It is these common challenges and experiences which not only generate many of the ethical dilemmas faced by nurses, but also form the basis of nurses' shared values and against which the topic of nursing ethics can be discussed.

In addition, nurses from the EU have the freedom to seek work in any EU country and a number of European directives mean that many nursing qualifications have common recognition. Study programmes such as Socrates and Leonardo da Vinci have created increasing opportunities for nurses to study abroad and a range of programmes designed to support and improve nursing services in the former communist countries of Central and Eastern Europe all mean that throughout Europe there is increasing scope for nurses to travel and work in countries other than their own. To a large extent nursing has always had a long history of sharing knowledge and experiences at both the European and international levels within a variety of frameworks. For example, the International Council of Nurses founded in 1899 represents nurses from diverse backgrounds and settings; the World Health Organization created in 1948; together with a number of European bodies such as the Standing Committee of Nurses of the EU (PCN) established in

1971; the Advisory Committee on Training in Nursing set up in 1977; and the European Nursing Group based on the Council of Europe with its wide membership and very strong links with the newer democracies of Central and Eastern Europe are all evidence of this tradition of sharing. There are also an increasing number of informal networks, such as the European Oncology Nursing Society; the European Association of Nurses in AIDS Care; the Working Group of European Nurse Researchers and the International Association of Bioethics, Nursing Ethics Network. A two-day seminar, organized jointly by the Standing Committee of Nurses of the EU and the European Nursing Group and entitled 'New European Structure for Nurses' was held in Niedernhausen, Germany in 1995 and enabled many of these formal and informal groups to meet each other and discuss the future organization of nurses and nursing at the European level. Since the first seminar, two others have been held, one in Madrid, Spain in 1996 and the other in Delphi, Greece in 1997.

It is hoped that this book, being prepared in the European Year against Racism and Xenophobia, will add to these efforts and aspirations and help to increase ethical and cultural awareness and knowledge among nurses throughout Europe.

The rest of this book

Nursing ethics is a growing area of concern and knowledge throughout the world. My interest began in the early 1970s as a clinical teacher in a major intensive care unit in a London teaching hospital where many personal experiences forced me to face the moral dimensions of everyday nursing practice. Since then over many years teaching nurses I was both moved and troubled by the stories which both students and qualified nurses recounted. What was particularly disturbing was that many of these nurses had carried their stories, not to mention a great deal of grief and guilt, within them for a very long time, feeling that there must be some weakness in them to feel as they did. Nurses, after all, just cope with the difficult aspects of their roles, don't they? This interest finally led me to launch into doctoral studies in the area of applied ethics and my PhD explored the nature of moral agency in the context of the nurse's role and afforded me the privilege of collecting over 400 critical incidents from nurses around the UK and in the USA, as an International Fellow at the Hastings Center, New York.

Since the advent of the new Diploma studies in nursing education (affectionately referred to as Project 2000) the study of ethics has been given a much higher profile in nursing curricula and consequently nurses in the UK are becoming better equipped to both deal with and discuss the issues and challenges posed by their practice. The same, however, is not true in other European countries.

In Central and Eastern Europe, for example, inroads into the subject are only just being made (see the chapters by Brykczynska, Northway and Reed in this text). In Italy, a government edict has recently ruled that ethics is to be removed from nursing curricula in all but a few Italian universities as it is felt that nurses do not need a detailed knowledge of the subject (Sala, 1997). The aim of this book, which is hopefully the first in a series, is to stimulate debate on the subject of nursing ethics, by nurses at all levels in their career and in all areas of practice. Although it is not possible to provide accounts of nursing ethics from every country in Europe, most authors have explored the ethical issues relating to various client groups from the perspective of the UK and at least two other European countries, so that a considerable number and variety of insights can be gained.

In the following chapter Win Tadd begins her discussion by arguing against Hunt (1994) who claims that nurses do not need a detailed knowledge of moral principles and theories. She claims that it is only through understanding these various approaches that nurses can think through the dilemmas that confront them in a rational and consistent manner. More importantly, it is from such knowledge that nurses' ability to mount arguments, justify their actions and challenge those of others, in cases of interprofessional conflict, can be developed. She provides an outline of the major ethical theories, principlism, deontology, utilitarianism, virtue ethics and the ethic of care, which influence moral decision-making in the Western tradition while acknowledging that there are many other approaches that might well be pertinent to nursing ethics in a continent as diverse as Europe. Finally she provides a framework for moral decision-making.

In Chapter 3, Astrid Norberg gives an account of the findings of a number of international studies in descriptive ethics which she has undertaken to explore nurses' moral reasoning in ethically difficult situations. The majority of these involved nurses from across Europe. After relating the concept of caring to relational, as opposed to action, ethics, Norberg describes first a study undertaken within an action (normative) framework followed by accounts of those which emphasize approaches based on relational ethics. In managing ethically difficult situations she proposes (as does Gournay in a later chapter) that nurses can be greatly assisted by systematic clinical supervision which can help nurses to understand patient behaviour and see them in a more positive light.

Norberg closes her chapter with an account of Logstrup's ethics. This approach, as well as combining problem-solving with the apprehension of a moral sense, also emphasizes the interdependence which exists between people and thus, claims Norberg, is an appropriate approach for nurses.

Christine Chilton's chapter explores the nurse's role as a health educator in France, Finland and the UK. After defining terms such as health education and promotion, Chilton gives a detailed account of the various approaches and roles which nurses can adopt in undertaking health education/promotion. Her major concern is with empowerment and the promotion of autonomy and she argues that there is a need for nurses to be empowered if they, in turn, are to be able to promote the decision-making capacity of their patients and clients. In doing so she draws on many contemporary examples from each of the three countries.

In Chapter 5, Rosie Tope and June Smail explore the ethical issues facing community nurses in Greece, Sweden, Finland and the UK and, rather than focusing on one theme, they discuss a range of ethical issues facing nurses in each of the countries. These include: policy development and the allocation of resources; balancing interests; patients' rights; justice and inequalities in health care; interprofessional working; confidentiality and adolescents; professional duties in the context of role expansion and autonomous practice; and competence.

Chapter 6 by Helen Crafter and Cathy Rowan deals with the ethical issues in maternity care in the UK, Italy and Iceland. The issues chosen for exploration include pre-natal screening; women's right to autonomy in pregnancy and childbirth; the role of the midwife, the value placed on women's autonomy and the value placed on the midwives' autonomy. The authors go on to draw comparisons between the countries at both the levels of policy and practice and postulate possible reasons for the differences.

In Chapter 7 Gosia Brykczynska considers paediatric nursing in the context of the United Nations Convention on Children's Rights. The countries selected for comparison are Poland, France and the UK. Before embarking on this, however, Brykczynska gives a very useful account of rights theory before discussing four of the most pertinent articles of the convention in relation to paediatric nursing practice.

In the following chapter Ruth Northway focuses on the ethical issues involved in the integration of people with a mental handicap. She discusses the right to community living, the question of choice and the problems surrounding the integration of this client group into health care. The countries chosen for discussion are Albania, the UK and the Republic of Ireland. Like many other contributors, Northway emphasizes that if nurses are to improve conditions for their clients they must become politically aware.

Kevin Gournay's chapter concerns the ethical issues which arise in mental health nursing. After providing an overview of mental health services in Europe, he centres his discussion on the issues of confidentiality, sexual and personal relationships, compulsory treatment, continuing professional development and issues connected with the elderly and mental health problems. He draws on examples and illustrations from Italy, the Netherlands, the Czech Republic and Eastern Europe and Scandinavia, comparing and contrasting these with the situation in the UK.

The subject of caring for older people provides the topic for discussion in Chapter 10. Jan Reed explores the issues of difference and distinction in relation to older people and asks whether these allow their particular needs and problems to be more effectively addressed, or whether they serve merely to create unhelpful divisions which result in discrimination. These

questions are considered largely at the level of policy formulation in Denmark, Bosnia and the former Yugoslavia and the
UK. However, Reed provides an illuminating account of the
relationship between the political and policy levels and care
delivery. She emphasizes the need for nurses to appreciate that
nursing care is provided in political and social contexts and
that these shape nursing practice in powerful ways.

Chapter 11, 'The Ethical Issues in Critical Care Nursing', is
written by Kevin Kendrick. After arguing strenuously for shared
decision-making in critical care areas, Kendrick goes on to
compare and analyse the very different experiences of Swedish
and UK nurses. Following this analysis he then discusses the
concept of ethical advocacy and the problems associated with
deciding who should determine what the patient's best interests are in any particular situation.

The final chapter by Verena Tschudin explores nursing ethics
at the end of life, comparing practices in the UK, Switzerland
and the Netherlands. The issues considered include neonatal
care, persistent vegetative state (PVS), care of the dying, organ
transplantation, euthanasia, advance directives and resuscitation. She draws particular attention to the effect of a market-
led economy on the value placed on any single life, the need
for skilled communication and the importance of virtues such
as compassion, empathy and courage.

Nursing ethics, as a branch of applied ethics, is both exciting
and expanding and it is hoped that this volume will contribute
to its development by exposing new vistas, visions and direc-
tions in what is an essential field of enquiry.

References

Campbell, A., Charlesworth, M., Gillet, G. and Jones, G. (1997)
 Medical Ethics, 2nd edn. (Oxford University Press: Auckland).
Colliere, M. (1986) 'Invisible care and invisible women as health
 care providers', *International Journal of Nursing Studies*, **23**(2):
 99–112.
Evers, G.C.M. (1997) 'The future role of nursing and nurses in
 the European Union', *European Nurse*, **2**(3): 171–82.
Hunt, G. (ed.) (1994) *Ethical Issues in Nursing*. (Routledge: London).
Sala, R. (1997) Personal communication.
Wilson, J.Q. (1993) *The Moral Sense*. (The Free Press: New York).

2

Ethics in Nursing

Win Tadd

Ethics in nursing

In the introduction to his textbook, *Ethical Issues in Nursing* (1994) Geoff Hunt decries the manner in which ethics is being introduced into nursing curricula throughout the UK. He states,

> many ethics courses presuppose that nurses have a need for 'help with moral decision-making' and that to satisfy this need they should be taught 'moral concepts' or 'principles' or even 'moral theory'. It is assumed nurses need yet another *procedure*, a framework of rules, which they can apply to the situations they encounter at work... In the case of ethics many appear convinced that a heavy dose of theories and principles carrying labels like 'deontology or utilitarianism', 'beneficence', 'non-maleficence', 'autonomy', 'quality or sanctity of life' will fill the moral void in our health care system (p. 4).

He goes on to claim that people entering the profession already have the requisite skills and that what they do need is the opportunity 'to freely examine from cases, preferably in their own experience, the conditions which create disparities between what their ordinary moral sense tells them and what they are expected to do without question'. He states, 'Yet surely everyone knows that student nurses do already have the responses of honesty, promise-keeping, respect for others, privacy, self-esteem and do understand these concepts' (p. 5). Hunt appears to take for granted that nurses possess a range of moral virtues and also that they seek to display them within their professional life but that the hierarchical and bureaucratic system in which nursing is practised militates against this. He states, 'To shed one's mufti and don a uniform is to be required to shed one's moral sense and don the metaphysics of procedure' (p. 5). The effects of working in such systems are well documented (Tadd, 1995) and should not be under-estimated; however, to assert that nurses have no choice about how they practise is not helpful and merely reduces them to the status of an instrument or object to be manipulated by others. Nurses, like junior doctors, administrators and other health professionals, must frequently make choices within the constraints of the system (Downie, 1984). Sadly some choose to be indifferent, rude, brusque or even cruel (Kelly, 1988; Laungani, 1992). An education in ethics is no guarantee that such individuals will practise ethically, but it can do a great deal to assist those who do have a moral sense and yet feel the effects of what can be an oppressive system. Take for example the situation when a nurse is ordered to lie to a patient about their diagnosis or prognosis. If nurses are to take seriously their role in protecting the interests of patients or clients in such situations, then they must be able to recog-nize good and bad ethical arguments, and be able to mount their own arguments as clearly and confidently as their medical colleagues, who frequently and with little justification assume moral leadership in addition to their appropriate clinical lead-ership. An understanding of the language, ethical theories and concepts and how arguments are developed is necessary to give nurses confidence to speak out and ultimately to demand accountability of those who give the orders.

Whose ethics?

Before leaving this discussion of ethics and nursing, it might be interesting to highlight a debate within the whole field of professional ethics. This debate concerns the relationship of the ethics of various professional groups to ethics generally. For the purpose of this chapter the debate turns on the rela-tionship of nursing ethics to the entire area of bioethics or health care ethics and there are at least two distinct viewpoints. The first view is that the term 'nursing ethics' is itself questionable as 'there is really very little that is morally unique to nursing'

(Veatch, 1981, p. 17). Viewed in this way, nursing ethics is classified as a subset of bioethics in much the same way as medical ethics.

The opposing view argues that nursing ethics is not simply a category of bioethics but instead '[it] raises serious questions about the aims of theory formation in ethics, the meaning of philosophical principles of ethics, the nature of philosophical solutions to ethical problems and the modes of work necessary for progress in philosophical ethics' (Jameton, 1984, pp. xvi–xvii). Sara Fry (1989, 1992) also argues strongly that nurses need to develop their own unique theory of nursing ethics.

My own view is that as the same ethical principles apply to all professionals involved in health care there cannot be a distinct theory of 'nursing ethics', 'medical ethics' or for instance, 'physiotherapy ethics', if by distinct we are referring to a set of unique moral rules or principles to guide the nurse's actions. There are, however, considerable differences in the practices and roles undertaken by different health professionals and this can lead to variations in judgements about the morality of various actions of the different professionals. Thus although the same ethical principles might apply to all health professionals, the implications of these for the conduct of a particular individual may depend to some extent on the structure, power relationships and conventions of the health care system as it is these factors which shape moral responsibility (Tadd, 1995). It is for these reasons that 'Ethics in Nursing' must be given a significant place in the nursing curriculum and be based on a thorough understanding of philosophical ethics.

It is also at this point when Hunt's views about ethics in the nursing curriculum need to be taken seriously. After gaining an understanding of what he terms 'technical ethics', it is essential that nurses examine the 'negative ethics' or the politics of the system which prevents them from doing what they have reasoned is the best course of action. Aristotle accurately linked politics and ethics and many of the ethical issues in European nursing can be traced to the way that health care is structured and the way in which the roles of the various professionals involved are shaped. It is only by extending the study of ethics to incorporate a political dimension that hierarchies and bureaucracies will be challenged and new systems of health care which ensure equality and afford individuals respect and dignity will be introduced. This volume is intended to contribute towards this goal.

It is also worth pointing out that if nurses wish to have a voice in bioethics or health care ethics, then pursuing a separatist approach may prove unhelpful and isolate them from the mainstream of ethical debate.

Approaches to ethical decision-making

Nurses face moral issues daily in their work and dealing with them is frequently, if not increasingly, perplexing and troubling. How exactly should we approach an ethical issue? How should we think it through? What questions should we ask? What factors should we consider? In one sense, each of us is faced with similar questions every day of our lives and indeed an important part of our early socialization involved us in learning that our actions are judged according to the moral rules that are widely accepted within our individual society. For example, as children we are taught not to steal, not to cheat, not to lie. A question frequently asked by children is 'Why?' and in order to justify particular moral rules different cultures turn to various sources.

Western approaches

Principlism

In Western cultures, the first source or level of justification is found in particular ethical principles such as that of respect for persons, the principle of respect for autonomy, the principle of beneficence or promoting good, the principle of non-maleficence or not causing harm, the principle of veracity, the principle of justice or treating others fairly. In turn, principles are justified by recourse to various ethical theories.

Many of the 'rules' found in nursing codes of ethics are underpinned by these principles. For example, clause 1 of the *Code of Professional Conduct* (UKCC, 1992), in demanding that nurses always 'promote and safeguard the interests and well-being of patients and clients', reflects closely the principle of beneficence.

Similarly, a clause in the Finnish *Code of Nursing Ethics* (FNA, 1996) demands that the nurse 'respects the patient's autonomy and creates for the patient possibilities to partake in the decision-making concerning his/her care'. The *Code for Nurses* (ICN, 1973), in one of its clauses, emphasizes the principles of respect for persons, respect for the sanctity of life and justice, 'inherent in nursing is respect for life, dignity, and the rights of man. It is unrestricted by considerations of nationality, race, creed, colour, age, sex, politics or social status.'

Until very recently Western literature on nursing ethics has focused almost exclusively on these ethical principles rather than theories, as not only are these easier to apply in day-to-day situations, but also viewing a problem from the standpoint of the various principles can ensure that a wider view is taken than would be the case from a single theory (Edwards, 1996). A major criticism of this approach is how to judge between principles when they coincide, such as when a nurse has to override someone's autonomy in order to either promote good or (beneficence) or prevent harm (non-maleficence). Despite this, the approach has much to recommend it, in particular its impartiality. This is not to say that an understanding of the various ethical theories is unimportant, however, as it is through these that ultimate justification is found.

A full coverage of the most influential ethical theories is not possible within the confines of an introductory chapter and for detailed accounts of the various theories readers are referred to the suggestions given for further reading. It is hoped, however, that an outline of the theories will assist the reader to appreciate the various influences in shaping policies and practices in health care generally and nursing in particular.

Deontology

This theory is most commonly associated with the German philosopher Immanuel Kant (1724–1804). It is a theory which focuses on duties and obligations and one in which the rightness or wrongness of an action is largely determined by the nature of the action itself. An approach from the deontological standpoint demands adherence to the principle of universalizability[1] and is stated in Kant's first formulation of the Categorical Imperative[2], 'act only on that maxim through which you can at the same time will that it should become a universal law' (Kant, 1964, p. 88). Kant's second formulation of the Categorical Imperative, 'act in such a way that you always treat humanity, whether in your own person or in the person of any other, never simply as a means, but always at the same time as an end' (Kant, 1964, p. 96), emphasizes the importance of the very broad and central principle of respect for persons in deontological theory. It is these formulations which result in a system of moral duties which must be fulfilled. If we consider truth telling, Kant would argue that because we are all rational beings, the universalizability of the moral rule which requires that everyone tells the truth is self-evident to a rational moral being and therefore truth telling is a moral duty. Also, the reason why we must tell the truth is not because it brings about good consequences, but because it is a moral duty. If I told you the truth because I wanted you to think well of me, rather than because of my duty to tell the truth, then I would not be performing a moral duty but would be acting from my own ulterior motives. In such a case I would not deserve any praise for being moral even though I have performed a morally right act. This demonstrates the emphasis which Kant places on the intentions and motives of the individual.

Kant links moral activity to being autonomous, as our acts are determined by our own rational will. When we act from desire or fear, or we unthinkingly follow orders, we are heteronomous as what we do is being determined by something or someone other than our own reason. For example, if I do not steal because I am afraid of being caught, then according to Kant, I am not acting in a morally praiseworthy or autonomous manner. Kant believed that each of us is our own moral authority and no-one else can dictate what our moral actions ought to be. In the same way, we must each respect everyone else's moral autonomy.

There are many aspects of Kant's theory which sit happily with our view of ordinary life. Clearly, most of us live by common-sense rules of morality and the wrongfulness of certain actions such as killing or stealing complies with the Categorical Imperative. The central notion of respect for persons is also very compelling as a central value in morality. Kant's theory likewise provides a secure foundation for the notion of individual rights which has gained increasing prominence in our everyday lives. Yet there are some problems with this approach.

First, there is no apparent way that priorities between perfect duties can be decided should they conflict. Imagine living in a country where civil war is raging. Your best friend, a resistance fighter, has asked you to keep secret the fact that he is in hiding near by. You give a promise not to tell anyone but a short time later the ruling militia knock at your door and you are questioned as to the whereabouts of your friend. The conflict in this case is between the perfect duties to tell the truth and to keep promises and as an agent you would have to decide whether to lie and keep your promise or to tell the truth (knowing that your friend would be shot as a traitor) and therefore break your promise. In other words, Kant cannot deal effectively with conflicts of duty.

A second criticism is that the absolute nature of perfect duties such as keeping promises or truth telling appears to need more justification than he offers. In the above case, for example, most of us would argue that saving a life is more important than telling the truth. It appears therefore that Kant has either overstated the importance of certain perfect duties such as lying or promise-keeping, or he has failed to recognize the significance of certain imperfect duties such as beneficence. This can be very troublesome for the nurse. Suppose, for example, that a female patient in her early thirties is admitted for investigation and, while talking to the staff nurse one day, tells her how before she came into hospital she felt so ill that she was sure she had cancer and that the thought of this terrified her as her father had died of cancer and, in the process, had suffered a great deal of pain. The patient then asks the staff nurse to promise to tell her about the results of any of the tests which she has undergone, as she is feeling so much better she is sure that it could not be anything too serious and she is keen to get on with her treatment and return home. The staff nurse reassures the woman and promises that she will tell her as soon as she hears anything. The following morning, prior to seeing his patients, the consultant informs the nursing staff that the patient has an inoperable cancer and that her husband does not want his wife to be told about her illness as, since her father's death, she has always expressed her dread of cancer. The staff nurse tells the consultant of her conversation with the woman and that, although she is unhappy about lying to her, she really believes that the patient will not be able to cope with the truth, at least initially, and that she may ultimately do better if she is not informed about the nature of her illness. Thus the perfect duty to keep the promise conflicts with the imperfect duty to promote beneficence and it is not clear how such conflicts can be resolved for the nurse concerned, particularly in this instance when it is unclear whether it is in the woman's best interests to know the truth.

In an attempt to overcome these difficulties, W.D. Ross (1930) provided a different account of the nature of duties by introducing the idea of prima facie duties. Ross denies the existence of any absolute duties, claiming that they are always prima facie or conditional. Unlike a utilitarian who would claim that the moral basis for an agent's duties must flow from the Principle of Utility, or Kant who claimed that it is the Categorical Imperative which provides this basis, Ross denies that duties have any such singular origin. Instead, he claims that duties arise from the morally significant relations which one has and that, 'each of these relations is the foundation of a *prima facie* duty, which is more or less incumbent on me according to the circumstances of the case' (Ross, 1930, p. 19).

In unambiguous circumstances, when an individual only has one prima facie duty then this becomes her actual duty, but where there is competition between different duties, only one can be actual. The dilemma of deciding which prima facie duty should be acted upon cannot be determined by the application of hard and fast rules. Instead it can only be resolved by carefully reflecting on which of the prima facie duties should be given priority in the prevailing circumstances. This decision-making is not simply arbitrary as some might wish to claim rather, 'each rests on a definite circumstance which cannot seriously be held to be without moral significance' (p. 20). Ross goes on to classify the various prima facie duties into duties of fidelity; duties of reparation; duties of gratitude; duties of beneficence; duties of non-maleficence; duties of justice; and duties of self-improvement.

At first sight this framework appears helpful to the nurse in deciding which duties she should fulfil. If we re-examine our previous case for example, it can be seen that the nurse would have competing duties of fidelity and beneficence. One which demands that she keeps her promise to the patient and another which conflicts with the previous duty and demands that she does not divulge the test results, although this may cause her harm. Although Ross's framework enables the nurse to clearly identify her particular dilemma, it does not offer any conclusive guidelines as to which duty should be acted upon. Even reflecting upon the morally relevant relationships does not really appear to help. For instance, it might be argued that because the nurse shares a special relationship with the patient, special because it is one based primarily on trust, her duty to the patient should override other concerns. But what is her duty to the patient in this situation? The woman has admitted her dread of cancer resulting from painful personal experiences and yet she has extracted a promise from the nurse that she will tell her the results of her tests. Should the nurse reason that the woman only wants to know the truth as she believes she does not have cancer and that therefore her husband is correct that such news will be particularly devastating? Or should she act on the basis that the patient really wants to know regardless of what the diagnosis or prognosis is, even though this will cause great distress? For if she fails to keep her promise and thus lies, the nurse–patient relationship, along with any future care, will suffer as the nurse will be forced into avoiding the patient so as to evade being asked difficult questions. From this it is easy to see how the claim, that Ross's system of prima facie duties results in no more than an appeal to intuitionism in situations where different duties conflict, can be made.

Ross's classification of duties offers no more help, therefore, in deciding or prioritizing conflicts between various duties than did Kant's and this is a major criticism of deontology. Despite this, however, the notion of duty is significant in nursing and has been since its earliest beginnings.

Consequentialism

Consequentialist theories, of which utilitarianism is probably the best known, hold that no action is intrinsically right or wrong. Instead, they are right or wrong according to their consequences. In its classical formulation, utilitarianism is found most prominently in the works of two English philosophers, Jeremy Bentham (1748–1832) and John Stuart Mill (1806–1873), and is perhaps best known under the slogan 'the greatest happiness of the greatest number' which under Mill became known as the Principle of Utility. This Principle of Utility states that actions are right if they bring about an increase in happiness or pleasure, or a decrease in unhappiness or pain, and that actions are wrong if they bring about an decrease in happiness or pleasure or an increase in unhappiness or pain. In the example cited above about the clash between keeping a promise to a patient to divulge the results of her tests and keeping an unpleasant diagnosis from her, a nurse adopting a utilitarian approach *might* reason that breaking her promise to the woman will cause more unhappiness in the long term as when the patient ultimately realizes the seriousness of her condition she will not only have lost trust in health professionals but will have been denied the opportunity to arrange her personal affairs and say her goodbyes to her family. This is despite the fact that there will be distress and sadness, even fear, in the short term. She may therefore decide that, on balance, greater happiness and less unhappiness will result if she tells the woman the truth. It should be remembered that an example such as the one above is precisely that, an example, stripped of its context and therefore some of its reality, to demonstrate how a utilitarian might reason about a very difficult situation. In practice, dilemmas are rarely as clear cut.

To determine the amount the pain or pleasure Bentham devised a calculus which considered factors such as intensity, duration, certainty, propinquity (proximity), fecundity (abundance), purity and the extent, in calculating amounts of pleasure or pain, and this was one element of his theory which attracted a great deal of criticism as happiness and pain are subjective and therefore virtually impossible to calculate. Bentham recognized that people vary greatly in their preferences and indeed on what they classify as pain. It was this recognition which led him to declare that so long as the quantity of pleasure is equal, 'push-pin is as good as poetry'.

John Stuart Mill developed and refined Bentham's work and the doctrine of utilitarianism. Mill rejected Bentham's notion that 'push-pin is as good as poetry' by distinguishing between higher and lower pleasures. Utilitarianism was eagerly adopted by many people in Victorian Britain who were concerned with developing a practical morality through which they could judge actions, thus utilitarianism greatly influenced nineteenth-century social policy. Utilitarianism was also believed to be just as each person's happiness (or pain) counted for the same as the next person's. As most individual actions take place within the framework of a community they therefore impact not only on the actor but also on the lives of others. For example, although I may derive a great deal of pleasure from playing my music at a high volume, my neighbour's peace may well be disturbed by my actions and if taking place late at night may deprive him of sleep. Utilitarianism demands that in any calculation everyone's interests are weighed.

Bentham and Mill are often referred to as hedonistic utilitarians as they imagined utility only in terms of happiness or pleasure (Beauchamp and Childress, 1994, p. 48). Happiness or pleasure, however, are not the only values with intrinsic worth and some utilitarian philosophers have adopted a pluralistic stance by putting forward a range of values which have intrinsic worth and therefore ought to be promoted. Other contemporary utilitarians (Singer, 1979; Hare, 1981) have argued that neither the hedonistic approach of Bentham or Mill nor the pluralistic stance of Moore (1962) are adequate to determine right action objectively. Instead they claim that 'what is intrinsically valuable is what individuals prefer to obtain, and utility is thus translated into the satisfaction of those needs and desires that individuals choose to satisfy' (Beauchamp and Childress, 1983, p. 23). Preference utilitarianism demands that in all situations we should act so that we produce the greatest balance of all the individuals affected, satisfying their preferences over them not satisfying their preferences. One major difficulty with the preference approach is how to deal with people who have morally unacceptable preferences, for example those who prefer inflicting harm or pain on others. The main response offered to this problem is that common sense, together with previous experience, are sufficient to determine unacceptable preferences and these are excluded 'on more general utilitarian grounds', that is, they would not contribute to the general good (Beauchamp and Childress, 1983, p. 24).

Another distinction frequently drawn is between act and rule utilitarianism or consequentialism.

Act utilitarianism

Act utilitarianism demands that an individual considers each action in isolation and should choose that which produces the greatest balance of happiness/pleasure/good (utility) over unhappiness/pain/evil (disutility), everyone considered. The act utilitarian therefore must look at a range of alternative actions and choose the one which brings about the best consequences.

One difficulty lies in the fact that determining all of the consequences of our individual actions is not as straightforward as it might at first appear. Imagine that my unfortunate neighbour is severely depressed when I decide to play loud music until the early hours. The effect of the persistent beat of my music is that he takes an overdose of tablets which results in a prolonged admission to hospital, loss of earnings and the breakdown of his marriage.

A second difficulty is that it is difficult to weight various types of human pleasure or satisfaction and, for that matter, displeasure, pain or inconvenience.

The major problem with act utilitarianism, however, is that it appears to allow any action whatsoever as long as this results in increased utility. This might include killing off ill elderly patients so that resources are available to the younger members of the community who contribute to a country's economic wealth. Torturing innocents, experimenting on prisoners, nothing appears to be ruled out.

A further difficulty is that this philosophy does not allow for any significant relationships which impose particular obligations and are a feature of most our lives. Such relationships might include those of husband and wife, parent and child, nurse and patient. Each person is to be counted as one and only one.

For all of these reasons most utilitarians have rejected act utilitarianism in favour of rule utilitarianism.

Rule utilitarianism

In rule utilitarianism a moral code is established by deciding which moral rules, if followed, would produce the greatest utility and the least disutility. Individual actions are morally right if they then accord with the general rules. Rules such as do not kill, do not harm innocents, do not steal, do not lie, do not break promises which, when followed by everyone, will generally produce more happiness than unhappiness.

Although rule utilitarianism addresses most of the problems that act utilitarianism raises, there remain some difficulties. First, clarification is needed about exception to rules, especially when one rule is in conflict with another. For example with our unfortunate couple above, a rule utilitarian must presumably ask, 'would the adoption of the rule with the exception (do not lie except when necessary to prevent breaking a promise) have better consequences that the adoption of the rule without the exception (do not lie)?' If the answer is affirmative, then the exception would be justified. However, rule utilitarianism does not overcome the basic difficulty which utilitarianism and consequentialism raise and that is that the majority will always tend to win over the minority, and when this type of reasoning is applied to allocating health care resources obvious difficulties arise.

Both deontological and utilitarian theories focus on the performance of actions. There is, however, another category of theories which takes as its focus the character of the agent rather than the actions which he or she performs.

Virtue ethics

There has been a resurgence of interest in virtue ethics since the publication of the first edition of Alasdair MacIntyre's book *After Virtue* in 1981, and these theories are now percolating into nursing. In a way this represents a full turn of the wheel as Florence Nightingale, responsible for the development of professional nursing in late 1800s, emphasized the importance of good character. For her, to be a good nurse one must first be a good woman and what constituted a good woman can be found in the qualities she expected of recruits into nursing. These included sobriety, loyalty, honesty and truthfulness and, according to Nightingale, these qualities formed the foundations of moral character upon which nurse training would inculcate the habits of punctuality, trustworthiness, personal neatness and obedience.

The claim of virtue ethics is that the application of principles or ethical theories of action depends on people being of good character and sound judgement. This is not to claim that there is no relationship between action and character, as clearly, how an individual acts often provides important evidence about her character. Similarly, specific character traits lead to certain actions, for instance when a compassionate person displays her compassion through compassionate acts. For a complete picture of morality, however, it is necessary to consider the internal qualities or characteristics which are essential for moral agency and which are at the heart of virtue ethics.

The main question in virtue ethics is, 'What kind of person should I be?' and has its origins in Ancient Greece. Although Socrates and Plato were both deeply concerned with virtue, it is invariably with Aristotle's account that contemporary philosophers commence their expositions. It should be emphasized that virtue is a complex concept as over the ages it has acquired certain connotations which were not originally present. For example, today, being virtuous implies that a person is wholesome, or trustworthy, or a decent sort who puts others before herself. It also has uncomplimentary associations, such as being a 'goody-goody'. In Ancient Greece *areté* or virtue had a very particular meaning and certainly had no negative connotations. Then it was used to refer to a person who displayed excellence in whatever they did. Contemporary notions of virtue such as benevolence, meekness or selflessness are in fact the antithesis of the virtue of classical moralists and the modern word 'virtuosity' might more effectively capture the notion of excellence evident in early Greek accounts of virtue.

According to Aristotle, a virtue is a habit (*hexis*) or disposition of character, concerned with choice, which is manifested in emotions; it seeks the mean in all things relative to us, where the mean is determined through reason; as defined by a prudent or wise man. These dispositions are not inborn or natural, but are chosen and acquired through practice and this, like the evocation of appropriate feelings, has implications for moral education which should focus on the development of the individual's character by inculcating appropriate habits or dispositions.

Virtue is not, however, merely a matter of acting in a certain way, one must also feel in appropriate ways. Thus, a virtue or an excellence of character is a settled disposition, and any action which displays virtue will also involve the display of some emotion such as desire, anger, fear, confidence, envy, joy and such like. For example, courage is an excellence of character (virtue) displayed in relation to the emotion of fear, while cowardice is a defect of character (vice) displayed in relation to the same emotion.

For Aristotle, there is no emotion which is either good or bad in itself, rather it is the state of character or disposition to display an emotion either appropriately or inappropriately which is deserving of praise or blame. What is necessary, therefore, is some way of deciding what is appropriate and for a complete understanding it is necessary to consider what Aristotle calls the doctrine of the mean.

Exercising a virtue involves the use of practical reasoning (reasoning which leads to action) in judging the mean between two extremes, one of excess and one of deficiency. Courage, for example, is the middle ground between cowardice, which is too little, and foolhardiness, which is too much. Displaying virtue involves finding the mean at the right time, on the right grounds, towards the right people for the right motive and in the right way. As to how one would determine the mean Aristotle has much to say, and he emphasizes both the role of reason and observation of those who possess practical wisdom. In particular he stresses three points.

First, one should try to avoid the excess which is most erroneous, so that for example in relation to modesty, shyness might be less evil than shamelessness. In this way one chooses the lesser of the two evils.

Second, everyone has a natural tendency to err on one side or other of the mean and therefore we must try to steer ourselves in the direction of the other extreme. If an agent has a natural tendency to cowardice then she ought to make a deliberate attempt to veer towards foolhardiness, thereby moving closer to the mean.

Finally, one must always be aware of, or on one's guard against, pleasure (one might wish to insert self-interest) because our judgement of pleasure is not impartial.

Despite his practical advice, Aristotle acknowledges that hitting the mean is extremely difficult and exact rules or comprehensive general principles cannot be laid down. It is more a decision which lies with perception and one has to be present in a situation to be able to judge or evaluate it. Only in this way can a person take account of the significant factors or values. Thus knowledge gained through experience which he termed *phronesis* or practical reasoning is important in knowing how to act in accordance with virtue.

In summary, therefore, according to Aristotle, virtues are those excellences of character which are settled dispositions of choice, in a mean relative to the individual, such as a wise person would determine, from the particular context, acting in accordance with practical reasoning or wisdom.

This notion of practical reasoning is important in Aristotle's account of virtue as it relates to the difference between the responsible actions of an adult and those of a child or an animal. According to Aristotle, the child or the animal are driven by passions such as hunger or anger, while the voluntary actions of a responsible adult can be influenced by his or her own internal monitoring. This internal monitoring or evaluation involves awareness of the possible outcomes within a particular situation; the awareness of choice between these outcomes; awareness of the different ends which may be worth either attaining or avoiding in relation to the possible alternatives; and a deliberate act of judgement involved in choosing and acting.

Thus, good people will have the ability to reason well about what is good for their lives as a whole and such deliberation will lead to the performance of actions in accordance with the virtues necessary for the good life. This aspect of reasoning is practical, social and political and necessarily involves others with whom we interact, influencing how we behave towards them.

For each excellence, there will be some specific emotion whose province it is and the mean is exhibiting the emotion to the right degree. If an individual displays too little or too much of an emotion then she is exhibiting a defect of character or a vice. Finally, there are no emotions that are good or bad in themselves.

It can perhaps now be seen why virtue ethics is of interest to those concerned with professional ethics but one must exercise caution as it is important to question whether it is possible, or even desirable, to identify or separate what might be termed professional virtues, from those that are necessary for everyone to live the 'good' life. Nurses, like teachers, bankers and shop-keepers, cannot leave their personal values at the entrance to their workplace and don an alternative mantle of professional values. The virtues which the majority of people come to accept during their early lives, such as honesty, reliability, compassion, integrity, courage, justice and the like, are precisely the virtues which should be expected in one's working life. Indeed this may well be part of the problem which besets many nurses, in that they falsely believe that their professional role makes demands on them which in their private lives they would not countenance. Lying to patients might be just such an example. The effect of this segregation of personal and professional virtues is a denial and disintegration of the self, which often results in feelings of guilt and alienation (Tadd, 1997). This is the point which I believe Hunt was making in his plea for 'negative ethics'. However, rather than claiming that this reduces the need for knowledge of philosophical or 'technical' ethics, to use Hunt's term, I believe it strengthens the need, as with this knowledge nurses are better prepared to argue their position and are less open to the criticism that they are responding purely on an emotional level.

Part of the reason for the perceived difficulties in relation to one's professional life lies in the fact that today the vast majority of people, including professionals, are employees of organizations and institutions and this creates various tensions and conflicts. For example, not only may personal loyalties or obligations conflict with those of one's professional role, but also there are often inconsistencies within an individual's role which seem to demand inconsistent courses of action.

It is for this reason that general rules and guidelines such as those offered by the Codes of Professional Conduct can appear to call for different actions when a nurse tries to follow their demands in a specific situation (Tadd, 1997).

It is presumably for reasons such as these that Aristotle himself highlighted the importance of context, when he said that only the baker can tell when the bread is cooked (1976, p. 120). General rules about how long an average loaf takes might be useful, but this dough, made into this size loaf, in this particular oven, burning that type of wood, may be very different from the average loaf. Nurses therefore cannot escape the responsibility of making judgements and they must consider how to do this wisely.

Also it emphasizes the fact that institutions must not only acknowledge the importance of individual virtues in their members, they must also cultivate the type of climate where people are expected, and are encouraged, to exercise those virtues. At times this might well include displaying a sincere disagreement with institutional policies. Thus, in the framework of virtue ethics, political awareness and action cannot be separated from a moral life. This again echoes the opening debate at the beginning of this chapter, but unlike Hunt, I believe that this further strengthens the argument for a thorough understanding and application of philosophical ethics to both the role and context of professional nursing, since through this political awareness can be strengthened. Professional judgement is not only knowledge of a professional nature, but also the practical wisdom as to which particular disposition, and how much of it, to display in order to achieve the particular good to which one is devoted.

On the question of which virtues nurses should display or cultivate, it seems essential that nurses are not callous or selfish, dishonest or untrustworthy, timid or cowardly. Thus, it seems appropriate to include in the list (which in the confines of a single chapter can be neither complete nor comprehensive), compassion, honesty, courage, justice and integrity as important virtues (Tadd, 1995). Also, it must be remembered that virtues do not exist in a vacuum and so the moral environment of nursing practice must be such that appropriate virtues can be both fostered and practised. This has obvious

implications for health care institutions and for nursing education in particular.

Like other theories virtue ethics is not without its critics.
Beauchamp and Childress (1994) suggest that virtue ethics alone
cannot adequately explain and justify the rightness or wrongness of specific actions and they rightly point out that individuals of good character are not infallible, they can and do
perform wrong actions despite being generally virtuous. Such
individuals can for instance 'act on incorrect information about
likely consequences, make incorrect judgements, or fail to grasp
what should be done' (p. 69). Thus, the major criticism is that,
as a guide to moral actions, virtue ethics lack specificity.

The ethic of care

A number of nurse writers claim that nursing needs a discrete
approach to resolve the moral dilemmas and issues which arise
as a result of the nurse's role and the current-day practice of
nursing. The ethic of care originating in feminist ethics appears
to offer a very alluring proposition for a number of reasons:
nursing is predominantly female and the ethic of care is
frequently portrayed as a feminine ethic; by focusing on care
not only are medical toes not trodden upon as it is claimed
that they travel the paths to cure; but also it offers nursing a
distinctive function within the health care arena.

Generally the ethic of care suggests that women approach
moral reasoning and moral activity in an entirely different mode
from that used by men in that, rather than relying on abstract
moral principles for guidance, they tend to focus on concepts
such as care, responsibility and interpersonal connections
(Gilligan, 1982). Certain quarters in nursing have readily
grasped these developments, for if it can be shown that a feminist ethic based on care does in fact operate, then as a largely
female occupation, whose unique function it is to care, nursing
not only has a theoretical basis, but also an ethical imperative
on which it can establish its claims to a distinctive role and
over which it can legitimately exercise supremacy (Tadd, 1997).

The ethic of care highlights the significance of interdependence in relationships where the specific situational and contex-

tual demands are given due consideration along with values such as nurturing, caring, compassion and empathy (Noddings, 1984). A detailed exploration of this approach is not possible within the confines of this chapter and readers are again referred to the suggestions for further reading. However, some criticisms have been levelled at the approach which are important for nurses to consider.

The first criticism concerns justification. It is important that when nurses are called to care, they know precisely what is expected of them. In other words that they care about the right things; that they do so effectively, and with skill; and also that they can explain and justify their actions. One important criticism of this approach is that currently the theory is underdeveloped and consequently it is very difficult to distinguish between the universally accepted notion of care in the everyday sense, and those occasions when the term 'care' is being used in a specific technical way as in philosophical writings on the ethics of care. This undoubtedly leads to confusion and a lack of clarity in the analysis of the term which makes justification of actions based on 'care' questionable by those who do not subscribe to a similar orientation. Merely claiming that each situation is contextually dependent and therefore certain actions may be wrong in one situation and correct in another is not satisfactory in professional ethics.

A further difficulty with this approach concerns how boundaries or guides to an agent's actions can be established. In their rejection of principled approaches to ethics, many defenders of the ethics of care appear to miss the point that often moral principles and rules exist precisely because we care for others and wish to live in relation to them, and without some rules and principles, such as it is generally wrong to lie, it would be difficult for society to operate in anything other than an inconsistent arbitrary manner.

The assumption, by many advocating an ethic of care, that principles are applied in a cold, calculating, abstract way can also be challenged, as can the fact that these proponents fail to see that they too are relying on principles, albeit different ones from those involved in more traditional approaches (Kuhse, 1996). For example, the importance of relationship could be claimed as a principle on which an ethic of care is based, and like other moral principles, should be defended on universal grounds.

In relation to this debate, at one end of the continuum impartialists argue that the only justification for preferential treatment is because close relationships impose particular types of obligations on agents, but that these are strictly limited (Rachels, 1989). At the other end of the continuum, particularists, such as those advocating an ethic of care, claim that the demand for universal impartial principles is an inappropriate basis for morality. Occupying the middle ground are others who suggest that there will be times when private and public morality will collide with each other and in certain circumstances impartiality will be overridden (Williams, 1981).

It is often assumed by those claiming that an ethic of care is an appropriate basis for a nursing ethic, that the demand for impartiality requires that an agent stand back from the situation and adopt a dispassionate or disinterested view of the issue or dilemma. However, this does not mean either that emotions have no part to play in any deliberations, or that one should assume that a disinterested position (one lacking partiality) is an uninterested one.

Suffice to say that intimate relationships are different from those which are role-based. For instance, husbands, wives, children and friends would prefer to claim that they respond to each other out of love, rather than because of some particular type of duty or obligation, whereas impartial and abstract principles are necessary to a public morality where we are involved with strangers (Broughton, 1983).

In nursing it would be extremely difficult to justify a morality based on particularity. Nurses should treat patients impartially by not showing favouritism, or giving certain people preferential treatment, but this does not mean they must adopt an indifferent or disinterested attitude. Nor does it mean that emotion plays no part in the delivery of care. In many cases, the nurse will be driven by powerful emotions such as compassion, empathy, even anguish, but these emotions are not dependent on the identity of the particular patient, rather they emerge from her reasoning that when another human being is suffering, he or she ought to be helped (Kuhse, 1993).

Because the ethic of care focuses to a great extent on women's experiences of caring involving relationship, responsiveness and co-operation there is a tendency to self-sacrifice, which has long been a traditional value in nursing and which should therefore raise alarms among nurses, as rather than being a force for empowerment, an ethic of care could reinforce the social and political structures which support the dominant relations within health care.

A further difficulty is the frequent demand for exclusivity and intensity of the caring relationship (Noddings, 1984). Although it may be the case that in the intimate caring relationships to be found within the family circle, receptivity, responsiveness and relatedness pose no difficulty, one needs to take account of the fact that nurses care for many patients and it is far from certain that caring to such an extent is either possible, or even desirable. A nurse cannot achieve high levels of intimacy and mutuality with every patient for whom she must care, not only because of the numbers involved, but also the average length of stay for a patient in hospital is falling rapidly, so that nurses have little time available to get to know patients. When the nurse cannot achieve the ideal portrayed, then she is left feeling inadequate in her relationship with patients (Kuhse, 1993).

Second, one might question whether patients want nurses to be closely involved to the degree suggested. Such intrusion could for example be seen as an invasion of privacy which has little to do with merely safeguarding dignity or promoting or maintaining the person's health status. Although patients may expect sensitivity on the part of nurses and a willingness by them to carry out their duties in a caring and considerate manner, there is little evidence that patients wish or expect a relationship of such intensity. What patients do expect, however, is competent care and to be treated as people rather than objects (Morrison, 1994).

Finally, there is a potential arrogance in claiming that caring is the domain solely of nurses. Caring is a human trait and therefore is just as likely to be exhibited by other professional groups, particularly in health care, where it might reasonably be claimed that entrance into this arena is motivated largely by altruistic values.

Regardless of the above limitations, therefore, one cannot escape the fact that for nurses, and all other health professionals, to display caring behaviours towards patients is a prevalent and reasonable expectation. No-one, for instance, would choose to be nursed or treated by someone who behaves in an uncaring, cruel or selfish manner.

A pluralistic stance

From all of the above theories it should be clear that none of them alone offers an ideal framework in which to view a particular dilemma or issue. Aspects of a deontological perspective undoubtedly have a place, for as health professionals there are some actions that nurses should never undertake and in professional life the concept of duty and moral motivation is of particular importance. The consequences of what we do as health professionals, however, are also important, not simply, though obviously, for the patient being cared for at a specific time, but also for their relatives and carers, other contemporary patients and, indeed, patients who may require our services in the future. Although the justification of actions is a vital element of ethics we should not forget that moral character plays a significant part in how individuals respond. Health care systems should be such as to cultivate the development of appropriate qualities and virtues to be displayed by staff whether they are front-line, for instance nurses and doctors, or those behind the scenes whose influence has far-reaching effects within the organization, such as managers and administrators. It is this realization which is slowly beginning to dawn on more enlightened organizations and is resulting in a growing interest in organizational ethics. Caring, although an essential aspect of human behaviour and a central value in enterprises such as health care, cannot necessarily provide an adequate foundation upon which to build a system of ethics.

Other theories and approaches

Having outlined a number of ethical theories on which to base moral reasoning, it is important to point out that there are many others of which space will not permit a discussion, for example, Niebuhr's response ethics, described in some detail by Tschudin (1994). Also, the above theories will be of less importance to people from certain other cultures than they are to those of us living in largely secular, pluralistic Western societies. For instance, in countries of the former Eastern bloc, an alternative to the individualistic approaches prevalent in the West, a 'materialist communal' approach to ethics, is seen as increasingly significant (Arndt, 1997). For other groups, daily life is closely related to religious teachings.

For example, for many Jews and Muslims the ethical decisions resulting from dilemmas in health care are approached from the perspective of religious laws. According to Jewish law (Halakhah), human life is sacrosanct, thus seeking medical attention by those who are ill is viewed as a moral imperative. A patient who refuses treatment (other than for reasons of futility or great suffering) is viewed as shedding his own blood and thus breaking Holy law. Similarly, doctors are obligated to extend their skills to those in need and any doctor withholding such help is viewed as shedding blood (Steinberg, 1994). These principles were poignantly emphasized in the family division of the High Court recently, in a case brought by the orthodox Jewish parents of a 16-month-old girl, suffering from type 1 spinal muscular atrophy (Dyer, 1997, p. 5). The parents opposed the proposed treatment recommended for their daughter. Doctors caring for the child planned to withdraw artificial ventilation via an endotracheal tube, rather than subject the child to surgery to perform a tracheostomy. In the event that the child, who was not expected to be able to breathe independently, suffered a respiratory collapse, the doctors did not believe that she should be resuscitated. In a statement to the judge, the child's mother stated:

> One of the principles fundamental to our religion is that life should always be preserved. Another is that someone of our faith cannot stand aside and watch a person die where their intervention could

prevent that death. In such a case, the person that stands by will subsequently be punished by God. Failing to resuscitate is equivalent to a situation such as this (Dyer, 1997, p. 5).

The judge ruled in favour of the hospital trust to allow the withdrawal of the endotracheal tube.

For Muslims, the Sharia' are the instructions which regulate their day-to-day activities and these are derived from the Qur'an (word of God) the Sunna and Hadith (the sayings and traditions of Mohammed, the Aimma (the opinion of religious scholars) and the Kias (intelligent reasoning or analogy to rule on issues not mentioned by the others). In Islam, the concept of family is of great significance and endeavours in medicine and health care are expected to serve and protect family life. Children are perceived as God's gift to a marriage and thus adoption, sterilization and abortion are unethical unless the woman's life is in danger or the unborn child will be seriously handicapped. Temporary contraception is acceptable providing it is safe. Because the interference of any third party in conception is forbidden, sperm and egg donation along with surrogacy are not allowed (Serour, 1994).

Although within the confines of this chapter it is not possible to consider every religious viewpoint which may prevail among the various countries in Europe, I hope that the above examples demonstrate how an individual's religious beliefs can shape their responses to questions raised by contemporary health care.

Living as most of us do in multi-cultural, multi-ethnic societies, what is important to health personnel generally and nurses in particular, because of the time they spend with patients and the intimate nature of many aspects of nursing care, is that whenever possible they should acknowledge that patients may not hold even remotely similar views about the ethical aspects of their care to those of the nurse. It is incumbent on nurses, therefore, to take the time to ascertain the individual's viewpoint rather than assume it will be similar to their own.

Steps in ethical decision-making

Nurses, like others, must realize that there cannot be a guaranteed formula that, when applied to situations requiring an element of ethical decision-making, will necessarily result in ethically sound or correct decisions. A number of very useful frameworks have been identified in the nursing literature (Aroksar, 1980; Seedhouse, 1988; Husted and Husted, 1991; Brown *et al.*, 1992; Purtilo, 1993; Tschudin, 1994) and all have much to recommend them. Below is a list of steps or stages, together with some questions, to provide a focus and structure in thinking through or approaching the dubious, grey areas which take up an ever-increasing part of our time and force us to make ethical decisions on a daily basis.

Be morally alert
People everywhere live their lives within a 'general structure or web of human attitudes and feeling... which forms an essential part of the moral life as we know it' (Strawson, 1982 [1962], p. 78). Recognizing and remaining alert to these feelings can indicate when situations involve a moral component. Thus, the first crucial step lies in recognizing that a situation or decision involves an ethical dimension or 'seeing with a moral eye' (Tadd, 1994, pp. 8–9). Ethics, therefore, should be recognized as an integral part of nursing practice and not simply an add-on after clinical, psychological and legal dimensions have been explored. This also means that nurses must remain alert and sensitive to the moral dimensions of their roles and this has considerable implications for the way in which nursing is taught.

Clarify the details of the situation
Gather as many facts about the situation as possible to avoid jumping to conclusions. Sometimes there is insufficient information, for example when trying to determine what course of action a patient who is unconscious would wish to take. In such cases certain assumptions will probably have to be made. At this point it is often helpful to try to state the case with as many relevant facts that are available as this helps in the recognition of both the central and marginal factors and in addition determines the decision(s) which need to be made. It is

at this stage that all of the interested parties should be identified as there are frequently more than are apparent at first glance. Also, it is worth considering the relationships between these various stake-holders including yourself.

Determine the possible alternative actions
The next step is to identify each of the possible alternative actions.

Evaluate the alternative actions
This is one of the most important stages as it involves evaluating each potential action by considering the morally significant factors in each of them. Potentially useful questions might include: which principles does an action involve? With regard to autonomy, one might ask if others would be treated paternalistically, exploited, denied informed consent, or denied respect and dignity. In considering non-maleficence one should reflect on whether anyone would be harmed either physically, mentally or emotionally. What would be the degree of harm? Similarly, with beneficence, one might ask whether a particular action would promote good, or avoid harm or perhaps reduce harm. In terms of justice, would an action result in someone being discriminated against or treated unfairly in any way? One might invoke the principle of veracity, by asking whether an action would involve deception, lying or a lack of candour.

Having identified which moral principles are involved there are other considerations which should be included. Deontological consideration would require that a person considers whether anyone's moral rights, such as the right to autonomy, privacy or dignity, are being denied. Thought should also be given to the obligations of each person involved which might follow from the particular relationships or roles which they fulfil. Also, one should give some thought to what would happen if everyone acted in this way. Does the action coincide with one's moral duties as prescribed in codes of ethics or professional norms? Utilitarian considerations would focus on the consequences of each action for each person involved and the amount of benefit or harm produced. One might wish to reflect on whether a good person (or nurse) for instance, someone with integrity, might choose a particular action. In addition the specific context should be taken into account. A further source of clarification and help can also result from discussing the dilemma with colleagues, other professionals, and friends and family. Often, by explaining a situation and describing the various options during an ethics ward round or patient conference, for example, one can gain insights about one's own values and the particular nuances of the situation. Sharing a dilemma or issue in this way can also reduce the 'loneliness' which frequently accompanies moral decision-making.

Make a decision
At this point one has to make a decision and having made it one has to live with it and whenever possible learn from it. Ethical reflection, like reflective practice, can lead to improved skills in making judgements. It is worth remembering that there are rarely perfect choices and with more time and more information most decisions could be improved upon. The improvement gained through spending additional time has to be offset, however, against the reduced number of options that might be available as time passes. Having made a choice it is essential that one accepts responsibility for it and uses the opportunity to grow both professionally and ethically, for as Tschudin (1994, p. ix) points out, 'making decisions can be difficult; it can also be exciting. It is certainly what real life is about.'

Conclusion

In ethics, as in any other worthwhile enterprise such as nursing or health care, there are rarely easy answers or quick fixes to the troubling dilemmas and issues which have to be faced. As we enter the next millennium it is likely that for all nurses, regardless of where they practise, such dilemmas will undoubtedly increase as technological advances become even more spectacular, resources more stretched and professional boundaries more blurred. Often, there is little time for deliberation and, like so many important decisions in life, they have to be made before an answer is fully available. This is why nurses need a sound understanding of relevant moral theories and

principles together with a decisional framework which is of assistance to them and which, over time, may become a pattern
for approaching morally troubling situations. Through the
study of ethics in both its 'technical and negative senses' (Hunt,
1994), along with its continual application to practice, nurses
everywhere will be better placed to clarify, defend and justify
the positions they adopt on matters of moral significance and
firmly ground ethics in nursing. It is important to remember
that 'right answers in ethics are few and far between, wrong
ones are devastating for all concerned. What is important,
however, is that as nurses we continually [and collectively] question our practice' (Chadwick and Tadd, 1992, p. 182). Sharing
the difficulties and exposing our deliberations to the critiques
of nurses across Europe, can improve our knowledge and
understanding of the ethical components of nursing and
increase our confidence in ensuring that health care remains
an ethical and humane enterprise.

Acknowledgements

The sections on virtue ethics and the ethic of care are reprinted
with minor editing from 'Nurses' Ethics', in Chadwick, R. (ed.
in Chief), *Encyclopaedia of Applied Ethics* (Academic Press: California). I gratefully acknowledge Academic Press for their kind
permission to reprint these sections.

   I would also like to extend my thanks to Marianne Arndt
for her helpful and constructive comments on this chapter.

Notes

1.   Universalizability is the notion that what is right for one person
     must be right for anyone else in the same position. For
     example, if I say that you ought not to lie I am committed
     to saying that anyone else in your position ought not to lie.
2.   A Categorical Imperative is unconditional, an order which must
     be obeyed as in 'Do X' and is compared with a Hypothetical
     Imperative which is conditional upon a particular end, for
     example 'Do X if you want Y'. Categorical Imperatives result
     in perfect duties which must be fulfilled without exception

and Hypothetical Imperatives in imperfect duties which are wider in that although they require us to pursue certain goals, such as the well-being of others, how the goals are pursued is left largely to the individual concerned providing they do not conflict with perfect duties which must take precedence.

References

Aristotle (1976) *Nichomachean Ethics*, translated by Thomson, J.A.K. (Penguin: London).

Arndt, M. (1997) Personal communication.

Aroksar, M.A. (1980) 'Anatomy of an ethical dilemma', *American Journal of Nursing*, April: 658–63.

Beauchamp, T.L. and Childress, J.F. (1983) *Principles of Biomedical Ethics*, 2nd edn. (Oxford University Press: New York).

Beauchamp, T.L. and Childress, J.F. (1994) *Principles of Biomedical Ethics*, 4th edn. (Oxford University Press: New York).

Broughton, J.M. (1983) 'Women's rationality and men's virtue: a critique of gender dualism in Gilligan's theory of moral development', reprinted in Larrabee, M.J. (ed.) (1993) *An Ethic of Care*. (Routledge: New York), pp. 112–39.

Brown, J.M., Kitson, A.L. and McKnight, T.J. (1992) *Challenges in Caring: Explorations in Nursing and Ethics*. (Chapman & Hall: London).

Chadwick, R. and Tadd, W. (1992) *Ethics and Nursing Practice: A Case-study Approach*. (Macmillan: Basingstoke).

Downie, R. (1984) 'Nursing as a role job', *Nursing Mirror*, **15**(4): 29.

Dyer, C. (1997) 'Doctors can end dying baby's care', *Guardian*, Nov. 20, p. 5.

Edwards, S. (1996) *Nursing Ethics: A Principle Based Approach*. (Macmillan: Basingstoke).

Finnish Nursing Association (1996) *Code of Nursing Ethics*. (FNA: Helsinki).

Fry, S. (1989) 'Towards a theory of nursing ethics', *Advances in Nursing Science*, **11**(4): 9–22.

Fry, S. (1992) 'The role of caring in a theory of nursing ethics', in Holmes, H.B. and Hardy, L., *Feminist Perspectives in Medical Ethics*. (Indiana University Press: Bloomington and Indianapolis), pp. 93–106.

Gilligan, C. (1982) *In a Different Voice*. (Harvard University Press: Cambridge, Mass.).

Hare, R.M. (1981) *Moral Thinking: Its Levels, Method and Point*. (Clarendon Press: Oxford).

Hunt, G. (ed.) (1994) *Ethical Issues in Nursing*. (Routledge: London).

Husted, G.L. and Husted J.H. (1991) *Ethical Decision Making in Nursing*. (Mosby: St Louis).

International Council of Nursing (1973) *Code for Nurses*. (ICN: Geneva).

Jameton, A. (1984) *Nursing Practice: The Ethical Issues*. (Prentice-Hall: Englewood Cliffs, NJ).

Kant, I. [1785] (1964) *Groundwork of the Metaphysics of Morals*, translated by Paton, H.J. (Harper & Row: New York).

Kelly, L.S. (1988) 'The ethic of caring: has it been discarded?' *Nursing Outlook*, Jan/Feb, 17.

Kuhse, H. (1993) 'Caring is not enough: reflections of a nursing ethics of care', *The Australasian Journal of Advanced Nursing*, **11**(1): 32–42.

Laungani, P. (1992) *It Shouldn't Happen to a Patient*. (Whiting & Birch: London).

MacIntyre, A. (1981) *After Virtue: A Study in Moral Theory*, 2nd edn. (Duckworth: London).

Moore, G.E. (1962) *Principia Ethica*. (Cambridge University Press: Cambridge).

Morrison, P. (1994) *Understanding Patients*. (Ballière Tindall: London).

Noddings, N. (1984) *Caring: A Feminine Approach to Ethics and Moral Education*. (California University Press: Berkeley, Calif.).

Purtilo, R. (1993) *Ethical Dimensions in the Health Professions*, 2nd edn. (W.B. Saunders: Philadelphia).

Rachels, J. (1989) 'Morality, parents and children', in Graham, G. and Lafollette, H. (eds) *Person to Person*. (Temple University Press: Philadelphia), pp. 44–62.

Ross, W.D. (1930) *The Right and the Good*. (Clarendon Press: Oxford).

Seedhouse, D. (1988) *Ethics: The Heart of Health Care*. (John Wiley & Sons: Chichester).

Serour, G.I. (1994) 'Islam and the four principles', in Gillon, R. with Lloyd, A. (eds) *Principles of Health Care Ethics*. (John Wiley & Sons: Chichester), pp. 104–16.

Singer, P. (1979) *Practical Ethics*. (Cambridge University Press: Cambridge).

Steinberg, A. (1994) 'A Jewish perspective on the four principles', in Gillon, R. with Lloyd, A. (eds) *Principles of Health Care Ethics*. (John Wiley & Sons: Chichester).

Strawson, P. (1982 [1962]), 'Freedom and resentment', reprinted in Watson, G. (ed.) *Free Will*. (Oxford University Press: Oxford), pp. 59–80.

Tadd, W. (1994) 'Ethics in the curriculum', in Tschudin, V. (ed.) *Ethics: Education and Research*. (Scutari Press: London), pp. 1–38.

Tadd, W. (1995) 'Moral agency and the role of the nurse', unpublished PhD Thesis, University of Wales, Cardiff.

Tadd, W. (1997) 'Nurses' ethics', in Chadwick, R. (ed. in chief) *Encyclopaedia of Applied Ethics*. (Academic Press: California), pp. 367–80.

Tschudin, V. (1994) *Deciding Ethically: A Practical Approach to Nursing Challenges*. (Ballière Tindall: London).

United Kingdom Central Council for Nursing, Midwifery and Health Visiting (1992) *Code of Professional Conduct for Nurses, Midwives and Health Visitors*. (UKCC: London).

Veatch, R. (1981) 'Nursing ethics, physician ethics and medical ethics', *Law Medicine and Health Care*, **9**:17–19.

Williams, B. (1981) 'Persons, character and morality', in Williams, B. (ed.) *Moral Luck*. (Cambridge University Press: Cambridge), pp. 1–19.

Suggestions for further reading

Edwards, S. (1996) *Nursing Ethics: A Principle Based Approach*. (Macmillan: Basingstoke).

Held, V. (1993) *Feminist Morality: Transforming Culture, Society and Politics* (University of Chicago Press: Chicago).

Kuhse, H. (1997) *Caring: Nurses, Women and Ethics*. (Blackwell: Oxford).

Thompson, I.E., Melia, K.M. and Boyd, K.M. (1994) *Nursing Ethics*, 3rd edn. (Churchill Livingstone: Edinburgh).

Tadd, W. (1997) 'Nurses' ethics', in Chadwick, R. (ed. in chief) *Encyclopaedia of Applied Ethics*. (Academic Press: California).

3

Moral Reasoning in Nursing: A View From Sweden

Astrid Norberg

Introduction

Moral reasoning, that is, the reasoning behind moral actions, is related to ethics. In the context of this chapter, a distinction can be drawn between normative and descriptive ethics. Normative ethics concerns questions about how we ought to be and act, while descriptive ethics concerns how we actually are and how we act. In this chapter the focus will be on descriptive ethics, describing how nurses reason in morally difficult situations. The basis of the chapter is the result of international studies into nurses' moral reasoning. These studies involved nurses in many European countries.

Caring

Caring can be regarded as comprising a task element and a relationship element. There is a carer who cares for the patent and a patient who receives care. The task element might concern, for example, the carer feeding the patient in a technically competent manner by ensuring that food is given in an appropriate way and contains adequate amounts or proportions of nutrient. The relationship aspect of caring involves the manner in which the task is performed, for instance by ensuring that the patient is treated as a valuable human being and is not degraded (Athlin, 1988).

This concept of caring can be related to ethics which focuses on either actions or relationships (Lindseth, 1992). In action (normative) ethics the question is: 'What is the right and good action to choose in this situation?' In relational ethics the question is: 'How should I relate to this person in this situation?' Virtue ethics is related to both action and relational ethics. It answers the question: 'How can I become or be a good person?', or in the case of the nurse: 'How can I become or be a good carer?'

Action ethics

Within action ethics reference is often made to general ethical principles such as those described by Beauchamp and Childress (1994). This approach presupposes that ethical problems can be understood as conflicts between different ethical principles and that these conflicts must be solved by deciding which ethical principle should be given priority in a given situation. The ethical principles that are most commonly discussed in health care are the principles of autonomy, beneficence, justice, non-maleficence, sanctity of life (sometimes regarded as an axiom) and truth telling.

An example of this kind of moral reasoning is described in a study by Norberg *et al.* (1994), where structured interviews were held with registered nurses in Arizona, Australia, California, Canada, China, Finland, Israel and Sweden concerning the feeding of patients with severe dementia who do not accept food. The nurses were forced to decide whether they should use force to feed the patients or leave them to die slowly without food. The study indicated that there was a connection between the willingness to feed and the ranking of ethical principles. Nurses who were most often prone to feeding the patient ranked the ethical principle of sanctity of life very highly, while those who primarily chose not to force-feed the patients gave a high ranking to the ethical principle of autonomy. All of the nurses stressed the ethical principle of beneficence.

Within traditional ethics is the idea that we reason in a rational and detached way which leaves aside the role of emotions as these are thought to cloud the ideal process of moral reasoning (Vetlesen, 1994). However, in reality, we all know that it is one thing to know how we should be and how we should act, but it is quite another to really be good and just and act in a good and right way. In practice this is because there is a complex interplay between what we perceive, think, feel, wish and who we are and how we act. I will focus on ethics in practice.

Relational ethics

Relationships occur mainly between people. Therefore relational ethics starts with the question: 'What does it mean to be a human being?' 'What does it mean to be affected by this or that disease and to care for that person?' Relational ethics in practice is founded on the carer's outlook on life. We may regard life as a neutral raw material that we can form as we wish, or we may regard life as a 'gift which makes certain ethical demands on us and feel it is important to understand and answer those demands' (Asplund, 1991).

Moral reasoning can be approached from various angles. I will address it from the perspective of the experience of nurses when they are in situations of ethical difficulty. How does the nurse react? Being in a situation of ethical difficulty is different from viewing a situation of ethical difficulty from the outside and reasoning about it without being involved in it. Being in a situation of ethical difficulty of course involves both relating to other people and acting.

By a care situation of ethical difficulty I mean a situation where the 'good' is threatened. One where we risk promoting the evil and neglecting the 'good'. I use the term 'good' as Murdoch did (1992) when she stated that good is good, and you cannot explain it to somebody who does not already know it. In other words, in my opinion, it is not possible to define 'good'.

Moral reasoning in nursing

Being in a situation of ethical difficulty concerns being sensitive to good and evil. We must be sensitive enough to perceive that there is a risk that evil will be promoted and/or good will be neglected. There is a need for ethical sensitivity, that is, 'a capacity to recognize the moral implications of one's actions in view of the vulnerability of others' (Lutzén and Nordin, 1995, p. 42). There is a need for us to be open enough to perceive and also to be strong enough to withstand what we do perceive.

Research findings show that carers sometimes cannot endure the emotions that are evoked in their contact with patients. Hallberg and Norberg (1990) found that carers of patients with severe dementia who exhibited vocally disruptive behaviour, that is, they screamed and shouted, sometimes seemed to regard this behaviour as an expression of an unbearable anxiety in the patient, such as anxiety for annihilation and separation. Despite their understanding, the carers isolated their patients (Hallberg *et al.*, 1990) and related that they could not bear the feelings of powerlessness and inadequacy which resulted from their inability to help their patients although they strongly wished to do so (Hallberg and Norberg, 1990).

In an attempt to ameliorate the negative feelings experienced as a result of being unable to help their patients, the carers reduced their contact with the patient. This kind of behaviour shows the close connection between the ethical aspects and the task aspects of caring. By learning more effective ways of helping the patient, carers can relate to patients or clients in a more positive way. It therefore seems reasonable to see ethics as an integral part of all care activities and ethical concern cannot be separated from concerns about care technology.

Another well-known example of this is the experiment by Milgram (1975) who, after the Second World War, wished to see how people would react when they are put into a situation in which they are expected to obey orders and those orders involve hurting other people. What happened was that some of these people devalued the victim and blamed the researcher (the order giver) for what happened. Accepting that they had contributed to another's pain or suffering seemed to be more than the research subjects could tolerate.

There are many phenomena in nursing care where we have to defend ourselves against truly understanding or appreciating what we are involved in and it is in these situations when we are tempted to treat patients as objects. Being in care situations of ethical difficulty therefore concerns knowing how to act. Some ethicists suggest that we can understand how we should act by going deeply into the situation. Our moral senses can tell us how to act. Murdoch (1992) is an example of this type of philosopher for whom moral decision-making is seen as primarily being based on perception rather than on rational reasoning. Other philosophers describe moral decision-making as essentially involving a rational and deliberate choice. We choose our values and determine our priorities and this implies a choice of actions. Hare (1961) adopts such a position. In his case moral reasoning becomes like problem-solving.

What we think about this question of how to act in care situations of ethical difficulty is connected with how we perceive the world. If we perceive the world as unrelated facts and values as subjective reactions to these facts, then of course we can choose from the smörgåsbord of values that various philosophies and religions offer. The basic question becomes not what choices we make but how we make our choices (O'Connor, 1996).

If we perceive the world as coloured by values, the task is not to choose between values but to attend closely to the matter so that we can sense and capture the values. Johnston (1978) writes about going deeper into the ordinary, looking with the eye of love, while Murdoch (1992) writes about looking with justice and love which includes unselfishness. Murdoch also emphasizes that it is important to be realistic. Freedom presupposes realism in that if we act out of a wrong interpretation of reality, the consequences of our actions will make it evident to us that we are not free to act in that way.

When physicians and registered nurses in oncological and medical care in Norway narrated about being in care situations of ethical difficulty it was evident that they emphasized different things (Udén *et al.*, 1992). Physicians narrated their stories prospectively while registered nurses narrated their stories retrospectively. Physicians focused on disease, scientific knowledge, preserving life, survival and the patient's best interests, while registered nurses focused on daily life, experiential knowledge, death with dignity, quality of life and patient autonomy.

The nurses emphasized relationships and care and the physicians emphasized choice of actions and justice. However, when these interviewees reflected on their narratives and penetrated more deeply their lived experiences of being in care situations of ethical difficulty, the differences disappeared. Common themes were: meeting death, balancing between being open to one's own and others' reactions and being sheltered, handling advanced medical technology and grasping care as a whole. Of great interest was the fact that the two groups disclosed different cognitive styles and types of rationality. The nurses very much referred to their personal experiences of both giving and receiving care, emphasizing the process of care. The physicians, however, referred to science and proven experience, emphasizing the result of care (Lindseth *et al.*, 1994).

In an earlier study, physicians, registered nurses and enrolled nurses in northern Sweden narrated their experiences of being in situations of ethical difficulty in intensive care units (Söderberg and Norberg, 1993). There were some differences in the accounts that seemed logical consequences of the fact that these professional groups have different tasks in care. The physicians mainly described the issue of over-treatment resulting from the difficulties in deciding about withholding and withdrawing treatment. The registered nurses primarily discussed their experiences of realizing which decisions might lead to meaningless over-treatment. Enrolled nurses more commonly spoke of relationship problems with patients and patients' families and the difficulties they faced in having to explain and defend decisions that they sometimes neither understood, nor had any power to affect.

It seems reasonable that the various tasks in care lead different people to experience different things. A closer analysis of the narratives disclosed similarities as well. Physicians, registered nurses and enrolled nurses all described situations that could be understood as tragedies (Söderberg *et al.*, 1996). Good solutions or outcomes were not possible and there were no easy answers to questions about the interpretation or the meaning of the situation. Patients and their families appeared as unjustly stricken victims. A difficulty identified in the physicians' stories was that of knowing what would be a realistic course of action, as it was important for them to perceive difficulties as well as realistic possibilities. The registered nurses predominantly talked about preserving patients' dignity in difficult situations, while enrolled nurses' versions described the difficulties of consoling patients and their families in situations without any hope.

The interviewees narrated how they created a silent space between themselves and their patients and the patients' families (Söderberg, 1997). They kept themselves and their values in the background to enable the patient and his or her family to express their experiences, values and perceptions of the situation without interference. They were attempting to be silent and attentive to subtle cues from the patient. Attention in a tragic situation helped them see, feel, understand how to act and perceive the possibilities that were available in the situation. This need for a silent space to enable an understanding of how to act was emphasized as early as the fourteenth century by Meister Eckhart who wrote about the relation between man and God. It seems that this is an analogous way of expressing the need for a deep involvement in order to be able to understand the demands of the situation.

By going closer into care situations of ethical difficulty, people are able to penetrate deeper, not only into the ordinary, but also into the unusually difficult matters. They look with the eye of love and create a silent space where the other can appear. Often this results in the discovery that they do not have to make a choice any more. This experience can be expressed as 'I saw', 'I felt', 'I knew'. Carers expressing these types of experiences often face difficulties in explaining their convictions. The experience is like the one that Martin Luther expressed as: 'Here I stand, and cannot do otherwise!'

Being in a care situation of ethical difficulty means acting in a way that individuals believe that they should act. As the Bible indicates, since the time of St Paul – and probably even earlier – people have asked themselves why they do not do the good that they wish to do and why they do the evil that they do not wish to do (Romans 7:13).

Wyschogrod (1990) suggests that people can learn something about the question of how they can act as they think they ought to, by studying those people who do that, for example, the saints. She discusses Christian, Buddhist and political saints and describes several characteristics that they have in common. I will mention a few.

The saints do not apply abstract theories to practice. They relate their lives to great narratives such as Jesus' life, Buddha's life or to a vivid picture of the society that politicians wish to create.

The saints have an open mind, they are deeply engaged with other people, that is, they are other directed. Saints are often connected with suffering. Wyschogrod emphasizes that this does not mean that they search for suffering, but rather, their open minds make them vulnerable and exposed not only to suffering and compassion, but also to joy.

The saints are directed forward. They do not go over their experiences repeatedly. They live in forgiveness, they forgive and accept forgiveness. Therefore they progress all the time.

The saints have a special perception of time. They experience time as the time left and not as that which has passed. It is their time, their due, the time they will have to take responsibility for. Therefore, it becomes utterly important how they spend their time. The saints know their priorities and can differentiate between what is important and what is less important.

The saints' actions hang together demonstrating integrity. They form a wholeness and express a message. The saints do not choose their actions as one chooses articles in a store. They do what the situation demands. This reminds us of what Murdoch describes when she suggests that when someone attentively goes deeply into a situation then there are no more choices to make and this means freedom. This freedom is, however, freedom to and not freedom from. In other words it represents an ability rather than a situation of coercion or constraint.

Wyschogrod describes saints as selfless, meaning that the centre of their personality is their values. As the Bible states, a Christian can explain it as: 'Now I do not live by myself, but Christ lives in me' (Galatians 2:20). In more prosaic words one might say that these people are well integrated with their values. This indicates that their moral actions are very much more spontaneous than is often supposed and not the result of moral reasoning as an example of detached problem-solving.

Although nurses, like most people, are not saints they can however learn from the saints. They can learn that the most important question is not what they do, but who they are. The question is less: 'How can I do good things?' But rather, 'How can I become a good person?'

Being in a care situation of ethical difficulty means needing support from co-workers. The saints certainly get support from their faith and nursing research has shown that support from co-workers can help carers to act in accordance with their conviction of what is the good thing to do.

In previous interviews experienced nurses stated that their decisions about ethical matters depended 'on the situation at hand' (Jansson and Norberg, 1989, 1992). In order to understand the meaning of that expression, experienced and good cancer nurses were interviewed (Åström *et al.*, 1993), and were asked to relate situations they had experienced in which it was hard to know what was the right and good thing to do. The situations described were interpreted step by step from two questions: 'What do nurses experience when being in ethically difficult care situations?' and 'What does the expression "it depends on the situation as to what I decide", mean?'

In such complex situations the nurses experienced many ethical demands, some of which were impossible, while others were possible, for them to meet. That is, the situations were regarded as either overwhelming or possible to grasp and the nurses either exhibited a type of loneliness or a form of togetherness.

When narrating about overwhelming situations the nurses mostly used the term 'one' about themselves and the term 'they' about their co-actors. When talking about situations which were possible to grasp, the terms 'I' and 'we' were mostly used. The most important situational factor in these narratives was whether the nurses had a group with whom to share their thoughts and draw on for support. If this was not the case then they had problems acting in accordance with their ethical reasoning and feelings.

In narratives about overwhelming care situations the nurses did not make a conscious interpretation of whether the patients' demands were also the ethical demands of the situation (Åström, *et al.*, 1994). In these situations there seemed to be distrust and destructive interdependence between the co-workers, and the patient was not seen as a unique and valuable person. In narratives about situations which were possible to grasp, the nurses made a conscious effort to interpret the demands of the situation and acted in accordance with their interpretation until a new interpretation was necessary. The interdependence among the co-workers was used constructively in order to care for the patient who was regarded as a unique and valuable individual.

It seems important, therefore, to change care-givers' perceptions of the patient in a positive direction. This can be done by providing them with the opportunity to discuss their spontaneous reactions to the patient and help them to understand the patient's sometimes seemingly bizarre behaviour. Hallberg and Norberg (1993) showed that carers, who got systematic clinical supervision and were able to discuss their patients and their own reactions towards them during supervision sessions, changed their perceptions of patients with severe dementia. They were able to see the patients more easily as human beings displaying behaviour that is a meaningful reaction to a difficult situation.

Moral reasoning in accordance with Lögstrup's ethics

Being a good person, however, does not mean that one does not have to reason in a problem-solving way. The question is how this kind of reasoning, which utilizes problem-solving, can be combined with spontaneous action. The work of the Danish philosopher Lögstrup seems to provide some ideas about a possible way of combining moral sensing with cognitive moral reasoning (Lögstrup, 1971; Bexell *et al.*, 1985). Lögstrup's account of ethics is ontological and relational. It verbalizes human experiences that are usually unconscious.

Lögstrup regarded life as a gift which has to be put to good use. Situations within our lives frequently present ethical demands which we must consciously interpret. Thus, Lögstrup described a human ethics based on a phenomenological analysis of life.

When we meet another human being, Lögstrup states that we may become embraced by what he termed sovereign or spontaneous utterances or experiences of life, such as trust, sympathy, openness, mercy and joy. These positive phenomena cannot be controlled. If attempts are made to produce and use trust and mercy, for example, then they will be destroyed and turned into mistrust and cruelty. What is possible, however, is to develop an understanding of how we can avoid preventing the occurrence of these spontaneous utterances and how to avoid their destruction. He also suggested that it is possible to create situations that allow for and nurture these spontaneous utterances. As we are part of the situation at hand and take part in the creation of ourselves, we should try to create situations that allow for and nurture these spontaneous or sovereign utterances. In other words we should participate constructively out of freedom. Every situation is both 'singular' and 'unique' at the same time as it is 'typical' and 'similar' and thus it increases our understanding of other singular situations (Armgard, 1993).

It is basic in human life that individuals meet each other with trust. Trust just occurs and Lögstrup emphasizes that this does not have to, nor indeed *can* it, be explained. What has to be explained are the situations where trust does not occur and the same is true for other sovereign/spontaneous utterances such as mercy, sympathy and joy. For example, when another human being is hurt, those involved may be engulfed by feelings of sympathy and mercy. This does not have to be explained. It is situations where this does not occur which require explanation.

When A relates to another human being, B, this means that A has power over B. A can, for instance, hurt or even kill B. B's life is in A's hands – in a literary or metaphorical sense. Equally, B has A's life in his or her hands. Thus everyone is interdependent, different parts of the same situation and of each other's lives. We have, therefore, to respond to this; either we take care of each other or we capture and destroy each other. To be interdependent does not mean that we lack independence but that we are free and independent when we accept the fundamental features of interdependence and subjectivity and accept our responsibility (Lögstrup, 1983). We have a free choice and a duty to act in accordance with the ethical demand embedded in the situation (Lögstrup, 1962). We must take an active personal part in the situation in accordance with our interpretation of the ethical demand and cannot simply remain a neutral spectator (Lögstrup, 1997).

When we are not embraced by spontaneous utterances of life and feel uncertain about how to act, we must consciously interpret the ethical demand that the other person represents. This unspoken demand is embedded in the human situation and Lögstrup emphasizes that the ethical demand is one-sided. We have to answer the demand without asking what the other person is demanded to do. The ethical demand is radical – we can never do enough – and it is unspoken. We cannot ask the other individual what it is but instead have to interpret the situation at hand. We can never be sure that we have interpreted the demand correctly, we simply have to take responsibility for its interpretation.

When interpreting an ethical demand, we sense the situation that we ourselves and the other individual are parts of. In order to sense, we must be open to receive and share experiences with the other person. This assumption that going deeply into a concrete situation means finding the good and right way of acting reminds me of Meister Eckhart's writing about a silent space (see p. 48). The interpretations of what is sensed are made against a background of prior understanding. When interpreting the ethical demand we are also guided by norms and values – important parts of our prior understanding, for example the norm about love for one's neighbour. When crises and conflicts occur, spontaneous/sovereign utterances of life might become verbally formulated and thus guide the development of norms and duties. The norms and values are in this way part of our outlook on life.

Lögstrup's account of ethics has been used in nursing science, for example by Saveman (1994), to reflect on formal carers' experiences of witnessing abuse of elderly people in their homes. Her interpretation of interviews with formal carers, for example district nurses, was that the abusive situations could be interpreted as situations where the sovereign/spontaneous utterances were destroyed and the carers had problems interpreting and acting in accordance with the ethical demand. They could not use their power in a constructive way. It is evident that Lögstrup's ethics cannot be used as a system of rules or principles that can be applied to a situation of ethical difficulty. It is, instead, an outlook on life and a way of reflecting on situations of ethical difficulty. Each individual must make his or her own interpretation of the situation at hand and take responsibility for acting in accordance with this interpretation. There cannot be any guarantee that the interpretation is correct. An open and serious attention to the situation and reflection about norms based on spontaneous/sovereign utterances of life are needed.

Interdependence

Lögstrup stressed the fact that people are interdependent and this aspect is very apparent in dementia care for example (Norberg, 1996). In interviews with carers it was found that those who said that caring for a patient with severe dementia represented meaningless work got nothing back from the patient. These carers talked about the patient as an object or as being socially dead. They expressed the feeling that they only 'work' in dementia care.

Other carers stated that caring for patients with severe dementia represented extremely meaningful work. They got so much from the patient. They talked about the patient with the respect deserving of a valuable human being and they appeared proud of their work.

It appears therefore that the perception of the patient is of the utmost importance in ethical nursing practice. Good carers have difficulty expressing why and how they find the patient a valuable human being. They sometimes use religious metaphors such as, '[when you care for the patient] you are caring for Christ. He is the one who is hungry, naked and sick' (Norberg, 1996, p. 105).

Conclusion

Finally, I come to a reflection related to virtue ethics. How did the good carers become good? In interviews, good carers often related experiences that could be labelled as broader experiences. Examples such as 'Before, I thought and felt so and so, but when my [mother, father, child] died, I understood. After that happened I see and feel and think in another way.' Thus carers frequently relate experiences that made them touch something 'holy' and that made them change their outlook on life.

In nursing, we cannot give students and carers these kinds of experiences but when they occur we can help them reflect on them so that they acquire positive paradigm cases. This is important because such situations can also lead to fear and defence and result in negative paradigm cases (Åström *et al.*, 1995).

Moral reasoning in nursing is therefore a type of problem-solving but it is one that must be based on carers going deeply into care situations, tuning into them, taking an interest in them and being affected by them (Vetlesen, 1994). This basic mode is an important basis for any rational problem-solving.

References

Armgard, L.O. (1993) *Anthropology: Problems in K.E. Lögstrup's Writings*, 2nd edn. (Mattissons Förlag: Lund).

Asplund, K. (1991) *The Experience of Meaning in the Care of Patients in the Terminal Stage of Dementia of the Alzheimer Type. Interpretation of Non-verbal Communication and Ethical Demands*, Medical Dissertations, New Series No. 310, Umeå University: Sweden.

Åström, G., Furåker, C. and Norberg, A. (1995) 'Nurses' skills in managing ethically difficult care situations. Interpretation of nurses' narratives', *Journal of Advanced Nursing*, **21**: 1073–80.

Åström, G., Norberg, A., Jansson, L. and Hallberg, I.R. (1993) 'Experienced and good nurses' narratives about their being in ethically difficult care situations. The problem to act in accordance with one's ethical reasoning and feeling', *Cancer Nursing*, **16**: 179–87.

Åström, G., Norberg, A., Jansson, L. and Hallberg, I.R. (1994) 'Nurses' narratives about difficult care situations. Interpretation by means of Lögstrup's ethics', *Psycho-Oncology*, **3**: 27–34.

Athlin, E. (1988) *Nursing Based on an Interaction Model Applied to Patients with Eating Problems and Suffering from Parkinson's Disease and Dementia*, Medical Dissertations, New Series No. 230, Umeå University: Sweden.

Beauchamp, T.L. and Childress, J.F. (1994) *Principles of Biomedical Ethics*, 3rd edn. (Oxford University Press: New York).

Bexell, G., Norberg, A. and Norberg, B. (1985) 'Ethical conflicts in long-term care of aged patients. An ontological model of the care situation', *Ethics and Medicine*, **1**: 44–6.

Eckhart Meister (1991) *Sermons & Treatises*, vol. I, trans. by Walshe, M. O'C. (ed.) (Element Shaftesbury: Dorset).

Hallberg, I.R. and Norberg, A. (1990) 'Staff's interpretation of the experience behind a vocally disruptive behaviour in severely demented patients and their feelings about it', *International Journal of Ageing and Human Development*, **31**: 297–307.

Hallberg, I.R. and Norberg, A. (1993) 'Strain among nurses and their emotional reactions during one year of systematic clinical supervision combined with the implementation of individualized care in dementia care. Comparison between an experimental ward and a control ward', *Journal of Advanced Nursing*, **18**: 1860–75.

Hallberg, I.R., Luker, K., Norberg, A. *et al.* (1990) 'Staff interaction with vocally disruptive demented patients compared with demented controls', *Ageing*, **2**: 163–71.

Hare, R.M. (1961) *The Language of Morals*, 2nd edn. (Oxford University Press: Oxford).

Holy Bible (1989) New International Version, classic edn. (Hodder & Stoughton: London).

Jansson, L. and Norberg, A. (1989) 'Ethical reasoning among experienced nurses concerning the feeding of terminally ill cancer patients', *Cancer Nursing*, **12**: 352–8.

Jansson, L. and Norberg, A. (1992) 'Ethical reasoning among registered nurses experienced in dementia care. Interviews concerning the feeding of severely demented patients', *Scandinavian Journal of Caring Sciences*, **6**: 219–27.

Johnston, W. (1978) *The Inner Eye of Love: Mysticism and Religion*. (Harper & Row: New York).

Lindseth, A. (1992) 'The role of caring in nursing ethics', in Udén, G. (ed.) *Quality Development in Nursing Care: From Practice to Science*, Health Service Studies 7, WHO Linköping Collaborating Centre (LCC: Linköping), pp. 51–9.

Lindseth, A. (1991) 'Ethics and meditation' (Nor.) *Dyade*, **23**: 26–43.

Lindseth, A., Marhaug, V., Norberg, A. and Udén, G. (1994) 'Registered nurses' and physicians' reflections on their narratives about ethically difficult care episodes', *Journal of Advanced Nursing*, **20**: 245–50.

Lögstrup, K.E. (1962) *Arts and Ethics*. (Dan.) (Glyndendal: Copenhagen).

Lögstrup, K.E. (1971) 'Ethical problems and concepts' in Wingren, G. and Aronsen, H. (eds) *Ethics and Christian Faith*. (Swe.) (CWK Gleerup: Lund), pp. 207–86.

Lögstrup, K.E. (1983) *System and Symbol: Essays*. (Dan.) (Glyndendal: Copenhagen).

Lögstrup, K.E. (1997) *The Ethical Demand*, Danish original 1956 (University of Notre Dame Press: London).

Lutzén, K. and Nordin, C. (1995) 'The influence of gender, educa-tion and experience on moral sensitivity in psychiatric nursing: a pilot study', *Nursing Ethics*, **2**: 41–50.

Milgram, S. (1975) *Obedience to Authority: An Experimental View*. (Harper & Row: New York).

Murdoch, I. (1992) *Metaphysics as a Guide to Morals*. (Penguin: London).

Norberg, A. (1996) 'Caring for demented patients', *Acta Neuro-logica Scandinavica*, Suppl. **165**: 105–8.

Norberg, A., Hirschfeld, M., Davidson, B. *et al.* (1994) 'Ethical reasoning concerning the feeding of severely demented patients: an international perspective', *Nursing Ethics*, **1**: 3–13.

O'Connor, P.J. (1996) *To Love the Good: The Moral Philosophy of Iris Murdoch*. (Peter Lang: New York).

Saveman, B.I. (1994) Formal Carers in Health Care and the Social Services Witnessing Abuse of the Elderly in their Homes, Medical Dissertations, New Series No. 403, Umeå University: Sweden.

Söderberg, A. (1997) 'The Practical Wisdom of Enrolled Nurses, Registered Nurses and Physicians in Situations of Ethical Diffi-culty in Intensive Care'. Unpublished licentiate thesis (Umeå University: Sweden).

Söderberg, A. and Norberg, A. (1993) 'Intensive care: situations of ethical difficulty', *Journal of Advanced Nursing*, **18**: 2008–14.

Söderberg, A., Norberg, A. and Gilje, F. (1996) 'Meeting tragedy: interviews with enrolled nurses, registered nurses and physi-cians about situations of ethical difficulty in intensive care', *Inten-sive and Critical Care Nursing*, **12**: 207–17.

Udén, G., Norberg, A., Lindseth, A. and Marhaug, V. (1992) 'Ethical reasoning in nurses' and physicians' stories about care episodes', *Journal of Advanced Nursing*, **17**: 1028–34.

Vetlesen, A.J. (1994) *Perception, Empathy, and Judgment: An Inquiry into the Preconditions of Moral Performance*. (Pennsylvania State University Press: University Park, Pa.).

Wyschogrod, E. (1990) *Saints and Postmodernism: Revisioning Moral Philosophy*. (University of Chicago Press: London).

Suggestions for further reading

Larrabee, M.J. (ed.) (1993) *An Ethic of Care*. (Routledge: New York).

Lögstrup, K.E. (1997) *The Ethical Demand*, Danish original 1956 (University of Notre Dame Press: London).

Murdoch, I. (1970) *The Sovereignty of Good*. (Routledge: London).

Murdoch, I. (1992) *Metaphysics as a Guide to Morals*. (Penguin: London).

4

Nurses as Health Educators: The Ethical Issues

Christine Chilton

Introduction

Autonomy, or the right of the individual to self-determination, while taking into account responsibility for one's actions towards others, is an ethical principle that has gained wide acceptance within democratic societies. The extent to which an individual has or can exercise autonomy is relative, as no-one has absolute autonomy. It will depend on a person's capacity to reason and make rational choices, as well as having the opportunity or freedom within one's environment to both make and act upon informed decisions. Creating and respecting the autonomy of an individual are two of the goals of nurse education and are values which are increasingly emphasized as the profession embraces developments in health promotion and moves towards a 'new nursing' philosophy (Salvage, 1990).

'New nursing' is a philosophy which has evolved during the past two decades from developments in nursing theory. Whereas 'old nursing' focused on the physical aspects of illness and task orientation, the essential feature of 'new nursing' is a holistic, interpersonal concern in which the nurse–patient relationship is seen as the key aspect. One assumption of this philosophy is that patients want to enter a relationship based on choice and shared decision-making. Putting this philosophy into practice requires an expansion of the traditional role of the nurse as expert and carer, towards one which encompasses the role of facilitator in health promotion. The holism which is emphasized in 'new nursing' arises from the incorporation of psychological, social and biophysical dimensions into the health model. This new philosophy of nursing has grown in popularity, alongside developments such as the individualized care and primary nursing and the wider social and cultural acceptance of individual freedom.

Incorporating the principles of this new approach into practice, however, is both complex and problematic. Recent nursing literature (Jewell, 1994; Trnobranski, 1994; May, 1995; Antrobus, 1997) describes the features of the new nursing philosophy and discusses the disparity between theory and reality. The ethical issues which arise in relation to this philosophy, the concept of patient or client autonomy and the nurse as a facilitator, will each be discussed within this chapter.

The World Health Organization (WHO) refers to health promotion as a 'mediating strategy between people and their environments, synthesising personal choice and social responsibility in health care to create a healthier future' (WHO, 1984, p. 73). Empowerment, or the creation of autonomy, is the goal of health promotion and in the Ottawa Charter health promotion is defined by the World Health Organization as 'the process of enabling people to increase control over, and to improve their health' (WHO, 1986, p. 1). 'Self-empowerment' is the philosophical basis of health promotion, and involves possessing the ability, authority or power to make decisions about one's own health-related behaviour and lifestyle without fear or coercion.

The development of health promotion

Health promotion and the new nursing philosophy have evolved during the past two decades, as part of the move away from the biomedical view of the causation of ill health and the associated dependence on medical care for disease prevention. These changes arose from the recognition that the major causes of premature death and disease were more often a result of social and environmental determinants together with individual behaviour and lifestyle patterns (Lalonde, 1974). As a result, the emphasis on both disease prevention and dependence on medical care in developed countries is being replaced by a more positive approach towards health and public health policies.

The role of lifestyles and the environment as important determinants of health status was further developed by the WHO, beginning with the Health For All 2000 (HFA) strategy launched in a declaration at the international conference on Primary Health Care, held at Alma Ata in the former USSR in 1978 (WHO, 1978). This vision was later transformed into a framework for health promotion programmes in the *Ottawa Charter for Health Promotion* (WHO, 1986). Outlined in the framework are five principal action areas: building healthy public policy; creating supportive environments; strengthening community action; developing personal skills; and reorienting health services. Health promotion has grown, therefore, from the formerly prominent health education by refocusing on building healthy public policy, but it still relies on these two components working together. There has been a tendency for the concepts of health promotion and health education to be used interchangeably. In reality they are quite distinct although nevertheless interrelated, as they both have empowerment as their goals.

Bunton and Macdonald (1992, p. 9) suggest that 'mediation, enablement and advocacy' are the 'process methodologies' of health promotion proposed in the Ottawa Charter through which 'people could begin to take control over their own health'. To ensure that a nation's health promotion programme safeguards the autonomy of the individual, that is, the freedom to choose and make informed decisions about one's health status, it is necessary to acknowledge that its two main interacting components, healthy public policies and health education, take account of the social and economic determinants of health as well as individual responsibility to maintain one's own health.

The World Health Organization has referred to health promotion as a 'mediating strategy between people and their environments, synthesizing personal choice and social responsibility for health to create a healthier future' (WHO, 1984, p. 73).

Health promotion may be thought of as a collective responsibility which takes into account the social and economic factors that determine the health status of individuals and communities. As a strategy, health promotion relies on two main approaches. Bunton and Macdonald (1992) explain that one is structuralist, encompassing political and environmental action and the development of healthy public policies. The second is lifestyle, which focuses on individual behaviour change and which is mainly concerned with health education. Both approaches interact with health protection measures, such as immunization and screening, and a useful and more detailed explanation is provided by Bunton and Macdonald (1992).

Building healthy public policy

This chapter will feature Finland, France and the United Kingdom as 3 of the 38 signatory nations of the Ottawa Charter. Moving at their own pace, these three nations are making the transition from traditional approaches towards health policies and health education that at present facilitate, to various degrees, the ability of the individual to manage his or her own health. Their governments have all recognized, at least to some extent, the contributions that nurses are able to make towards the health of their nations through health promotion and health education.

Since 1982, Finland has been the pilot country for the WHO's HFA strategy development and in 1985 it became the first country in Europe to issue a national strategy for HFA. This has a strong emphasis on lifestyles and combines both behavioural and public policy approaches to health promotion and disease prevention. However, the deep economic recession of the early 1990s, leading to high unemployment, has slowed down the implementation of some targeted projects, especially those aimed at the adult population through occupational health services and those planned to reduce the socio-economic differences in health (Eskola, 1995).

The United Kingdom, in accordance with the principles of WHO's HFA strategy (WHO, 1985), issued four national health strategy documents *The Health of the Nation* (Department of Health, 1992). The strategy for England emphasizing the need for individual lifestyle changes of identified high risk groups and the meeting of specific targets has been criticized for not adequately taking into account the social and economic factors that determine health (Hagard, 1995).

In France, the biomedical model remains dominant in the perception of the general public, professionals and policy-makers. In the literature, public health issues tend to be viewed in epidemiological terms rather than as an evaluation of health promotion interventions. There is relatively little discourse which defines and analyses the concepts of health promotion and health education, as is apparent in the United Kingdom and Finnish literature. However, on a practical level, a variety of health education and health promotion structures exist at the state, municipality public sector and the voluntary sector levels so that these twin concepts are brought together in health service action. Since 1994, health priorities and measurable objectives have been identified and a framework for a compre-hensive and co-ordinated health promotion programme is being developed (Demeulemeester and Baudier, 1995).These will be transmitted through existing health promotion, health educa-tion and health service structures within the public and volun-tary sectors at regional and local levels (Tessier *et al.*, 1996).

In reality, as each nation moves at its own pace towards the achievement of HFA, ethical issues arise in relation to the autonomy of patients and clients and the extent to which nurses are empowered to enact their role as health educators. These issues, in the context of Finland, France and the United Kingdom, will provide the main focus of this chapter. It is necessary first, however, to consider the concept of health.

Health

Health is an ambiguous and subjectively understood concept whose range of meanings stretch from that of the narrow bio-medical model to one that is broad and holistic. Nordenfelt, in his book *Quality of Life, Health and Happiness* (1993), gives a detailed analysis of the range of philosophical accounts of health, disease and illness, commencing with Boorse's narrow biostat-istical theory and concluding with a detailed description of 'subjective health'. What Nordenfelt's work demonstrates is that health is an 'essentially contested concept' (Gallie, 1955–56) which means that whenever statements about terms such as health are made questions of value are raised which seem to prevent agreement on a conclusive definition or indeed appropriate usage of the terms. According to Gallie, essentially contested concepts have three main characteristics. First, they are 'appraisive' (p. 171) in the sense of not only naming the concept but also ascribing a value with respect to it. Second, essentially contested concepts are 'internally complex' (pp. 171–2), in that their characterizations entail reference to several dimensions. Third, an essentially contested concept is 'open' (p. 172) so that participants in the debate are able to interpret it in a number of different ways. These difficulties have led to problems in gaining agreement on what constitutes health with the result that proponents frequently talk at cross purposes. One way to overcome these problems is to accept that there is only one concept of health but many different conceptions of it (Lindley, 1986). 'A conception is a particular interpretation or analysis of a concept... An adequate conception must fall within the scope of the basic concept' (Lindley, 1986, p. 3) so that whenever an abstract concept such as health is expanded with different content, it can be said that there is a conception of the concept. An illustration may help to clarify this particular use of these terms. Imagine, for example, two individuals who have acquired the concept of a dog, an animal with four legs, a tail and which barks. However, if one had experienced only pit bull terriers and the other only chihuahuas, their individual conceptions of 'dog' would be very different (Tadd, 1995). In the case of health, therefore, its definitions are based on value judgements, whether these are the goals and beliefs of health professionals or the 'common-sense' views of lay individuals. A gap between professional and lay concepts of health can give rise to problems of communication and co-operation. Thus an open-minded approach to determining people's views of what it means to be healthy, or to lead a healthy lifestyle, is needed by health professionals.

Health definitions have 'polarity', that is, they can range anywhere on a continuum between a negative definition, as in health being the absence of disease or illness, to one that is positive, such as health as a state of well-being. The World Health Organization acknowledges that health is a holistic and dynamic concept of interdependent, internal dimensions which act together or separately and are affected by the social, economic and physical environment. Its own historical and rather idealistic definition of health as 'a state of complete physical, mental and social well-being, and not merely the absence of disease or infirmity' (WHO, 1948, p. 1) has, since its original appearance, undergone further development.

As proposed by WHO (1984), being healthy should have a purpose and instrumental value as a resource, rather than simply being an end in itself of perfect well-being. At the 30th World Health Assembly in 1978 the WHO adopted a resolution that the main social goal of health according to the WHO 'should be the attainment by all the people of the world by the year 2000, of a level of health that will permit them to lead a socially and economically productive life' (WHO, 1985, p. 1). As a result of this resolution, a unanimous commitment to the HFA strategy was made in the Alma Ata declaration (WHO, 1978). Thus the achievement of health ought to be a means to an end which exists within a political context and relies upon healthy public policies at national and local government levels.

From a global view of health to one that is meaningful to the individual, it can be seen that no single, universal definition of health exists. However, while it may be impossible to predict an individual's view of health, differing views associated with social class and cultural groups should be acknowledged. These views often concern beliefs about the amount of choice and power available to individuals and these in turn shape the decisions individuals make which influence or determine their lives and health.

Health education and the role of the nurse

Health promotion and health education are integral to nursing, but there has been a tendency for nurses to use the terms interchangeably (Latter *et al.*, 1992). They are, as has been discussed, quite distinct, although necessarily interrelated, activities with empowerment as their mutual goal.

Health education is a planned activity intended to provide knowledge and assist understanding about health issues as well as enabling people to incorporate their health choices into

their own lives. Current approaches invite the active participation of individuals and communities in all decision-making.

As Delaney (1994) suggests, health education is the most
easily distinguishable element of health promotion in which
nurses and midwives participate. In the majority of cases health
education undertaken by nurses and midwives focuses on the
individual and Delaney (1994) defends this by arguing that it
is unreasonable '...to expect any group or individual to operate
at all levels of health promotion'. It is for these reasons that
this chapter will focus on the narrower role of the nurse as a
health educator. In this role a range of individually focused
approaches can be used, each defined according to their goals,
activities and underlying values. These approaches may be
used singly or in combination and Ewles and Simnett (1992)
suggest that there is no one 'right' approach, but rather the
choice should depend on an assessment of individual/commu-
nity needs as well as the values and code of conduct of the
health professional. It must be emphasized that, in all cases,
health education should involve voluntary change and not have
to rely on persuasion, coercion or indoctrination.

Behaviour change approach

In this approach individuals are encouraged to take responsibility for their health by changing health-damaging attitudes
and behaviours in favour of healthier lifestyles as defined by
experts. Acting in a manner perceived to be in the best interests of the individual and with the aim of achieving compliance, persuasive interventions are frequently used. These may
include one-to-one advice, information and mass media
campaigns. The powerful persuasiveness of health-damaging
influences such as cigarette advertising is frequently cited as
a justification and these interventions often target behaviours
such as smoking, excessive drinking, lack of exercise, unhealthy
eating and unsafe sex. For example, *The Health of the Nation*
(Department of Health, 1992) strategy for England includes
targets such as a reduction in the number of people who
smoke cigarettes and encouraging individuals to adopt healthy
behaviours is proposed as a legitimate activity of health profes-

sionals. One problem with this approach is that a failure to achieve the targets set can result in victim blaming while the social and economic factors that affect people's choices and decisions are ignored. A further problem is that such strategies place little value on individual autonomy and can be seen as moralizing.

Educational approach

In this approach the aim is to improve knowledge, develop skills for healthy living and ensure understanding so that individuals can make an informed choice about their health behaviour. The approach respects the right of individuals to choose their own health behaviours. Information is provided through one-to-one teaching or in small discussion groups, with the content often being influenced by clients' expressed needs. In addition individuals are helped to explore their values and attitudes and to carry out their own decisions. The approach is particularly suitable for antenatal and child care, school and workplace programmes as well as individual patient education concerning specific disease, treatment and rehabilitation procedures. Written information is often given to these individuals and their families to read; however, patient/client education has been found to more effective and acceptable when it is designed specifically to meet the needs of those concerned through follow-up discussions which provide opportunities for asking questions and receiving supportive explanations from nurses and midwives.

A review of the literature indicates that this approach is used in Finland for family training and support of couples in their transition to parenthood (Vehvilainen-Julkunen, 1995) as well as to achieve active and responsible self-care in adolescent diabetics (Kyngas and Hentinen, 1995). In France, Marty and Macaux (1997) have adopted an educational format for written information offered to breast cancer patients undergoing surgery. Included in this information package is advice on the nurse's role in health education and the women are invited to seek further explanations from nursing staff. Through group discussions and the publication of a newsletter, a team of occupational health nurses in France have been able to successfully advise on the prevention of chemical hazards (Manicot, 1991). In the United Kingdom, this approach, often termed teaching and information giving, has been identified in the surveys of Davis (1995), McBride (1994) and Noble (1991).

Client-centred approach

This approach relies on professionals working as equal partners with individuals to help them identify their concerns, the aspects of their lives that require change and the choices that are available to them. Individuals are then helped to gain the skills of informed decision-making and the confidence to act upon their decisions so that they can take control of their lives and health. The approach is centred on the individual and, with its goal of self-empowerment of the patient or client, may involve one-to-one counselling. In Finland, for example, an examination of the client-centred approach demonstrated that the relationships between mothers and public health nurses during visits to health clinics supported self-confidence and participation through negotiation, information sharing and advising (Vehviläinen-Julkunen, 1992).

The nurse's role as a health educator can be described according to two main styles of intervention ranging from authoritarian (nurse as expert) to negotiator (nurse as facilitator) (Ewles and Simnett, 1992). The ethical implications of these roles are discussed below.

Nurse as expert

This traditional image of the nursing role is one in which paternalistic action features strongly. It tends to be popular within the health care professions as it is so clearly defined. The nurse is a source of knowledge who provides information, advice and guidance to clients or patients in order to bring about a change in their behaviour which will include taking responsibility for their own health. The chosen activities rely on the nurse's assessment of the need for change, the

appropriateness of the individual's lifestyle and the most effective means of communication. It results in a one-way flow of
information which may not always be relevant to an individual's
particular needs or circumstances. The acceptance of the health
message may rely on the nurse's status, her credibility and
trustworthiness. However, persuasion or coercion may result if
nurses impose their own values, solutions or instructions as a
way of dealing with a client's problems. This necessarily denies
the individual the right to freely choose their health-related
behaviours and therefore is unethical.

The model ignores the social and environmental dimensions
of health and as with the behaviour change approach discussed
above, assumes that individuals have equal resources thereby
ignoring the complex relationship between individual behaviour and social and environmental factors.

By the patient or client adopting a passive role, compliance
is expected. This can be reassuring to those who are vulnerable, such as children or those who are very ill and have rather
limited levels of autonomy. The disadvantage of such an approach
is that by fostering dependency on medical knowledge, rather
than encouraging autonomy, individuals neither develop the
ability, nor acquire the resources, to accept responsibility for
their own decisions and actions. Although adoption of the role
of expert has been successful in patient education when it is
necessary to avoid distress, such as providing information prior
to or after surgical or investigatory procedures, it has not been
effective in changing the long-held, health-related behaviours
which affect lifestyle. It is these which often pose the greatest
challenge for nurses working in primary health care settings
such as schools and workplaces. The ability to communicate is
simply not enough. It is necessary to take into account not only
an individual's stage of development and emotional condition,
but also his or her social and cultural background.

Ethical issues also arise because of the assumption that
everyone has equal resources and abilities to comply with the
directives given. When compliance is not achieved then victim
blaming may occur, even if it is not deliberately intended. In
other words, individuals are held solely responsible for the
factors which have put them at a disadvantage, but over which
they may have no control. Similarly, health problems attributed

to particular groups may also lead to victim blaming. Perhaps nowhere was this more obvious than in the early days of the AIDS outbreak. Mothers and fathers attending family training in Finland evaluated the role of the public health nurse and midwife as an important expert (Vehviläinen-Julkunen, 1995).

Nurse as a facilitator

In adopting this role, the nurse seeks to enhance the autonomy of the patient or client and it is this image which many nurses aspire to within the new nursing philosophy. The model lies comfortably with the client-centred and educational approaches that invite the participation of individuals. Examples are cited in the literature by Vehviläinen-Julkunen (1992) and Kyngas and Hentinen (1995). In this role, nurses utilize activities and methods that are planned in consultation with the individual, using stages similar to those of the nursing process. Through the process of negotiation, a careful assessment of the individual's needs are made.

As a facilitator, the nurse should enact her role with warmth and empathy, building confidence, sharing skills and knowledge and encouraging the individual to enter into a relationship of trust and openness. Through the individual's choice to actively participate in negotiation and shared decision-making, their autonomy is not only respected, but may also be enhanced. In this way individuals learn to trust their own judgement.

The nurse is required to respect informed decisions made by the individual, even if these are not ones with which she would concur or that will lead to a healthy outcome. This can create a dilemma for nurses whose intent is to 'do good', where 'good' is defined in some sense of 'health'.

Nurses aspiring to the role of facilitator must be aware that although educational approaches aim to enhance autonomy by providing knowledge that will enable the individual to make an informed choice, unlike client-centred approaches, they may ignore both the restrictions that social and economic factors place on voluntary behaviour change and the complex nature of health-related decision-making. Self-empowerment enables individuals to act in ways that influence these factors within their own communities.

The new nursing philosophy, with its aspirations for self-empowerment, assumes that patients or clients want to be active participants but this should be seen as their choice. There are of course various types and degrees of participation which may vary over time according to the needs of the individual. If nurses are inflexible and assume that all patients or clients should be encouraged to become active participants in decision-making, regardless of its appropriateness to the particular individual, then coercion and compliance may occur. To avoid this, patients and clients should be asked if they wish to become involved (Waterworth and Luker, 1990). On the other hand, the provision of information is a fundamental need and according to European Union regulations, it is a legal right. Furthermore, there is an ethical obligation that the quality of information provided should enable individuals to understand the medical aspects of their condition or state of health and to participate in decisions which will have consequences on their well-being (Posko, 1993).

In the UK nursing literature descriptions and discussions of this style of role enactment can be found in the work of Waterworth and Luker (1990), Jewell (1994) and Trnobranski (1994) but similar topics are not apparent in the Finnish and French literature.

The need to empower nurses in Finland, France and the United Kingdom

To achieve the goal of self-empowerment the relationship of patients and clients with the nurse must undergo a transition of power and control by moving away from the nurse's traditional role as expert to that of facilitator. The patient's or client's autonomy is enhanced, while the nurse's authority, in her role as a health educator, is reduced. However, to fulfil a professional role that facilitates empowerment and encourages collaboration and active participation in both self-care and decision-making, nurses need to have both the authority and therefore the autonomy necessary to enable patients and clients to enact the decisions they have made.

Finland

Finland has a long and distinguished history of public health nursing providing an extensive service in municipal health centres. Although reforms over the years have altered this service, the public health nurse, together with the doctor, still remains a key person in primary health care as Tope and Smail discuss in the following chapter. She is able to work directly with clients and has the authority to initiate contacts and consult expert members of the health care team (Siivola and Martikainen, 1990). Public health nurses undergo four and a half years of education (including three years of general nursing education), but the authors admit that 'developing the quality and content of public health nursing continues to pose an educational and managerial challenge' (p. 107). The role of health educator is also incorporated into the role of registered nurses working in the hospital sector.

Within the hospital setting in Finland, gaps have been identified between the government's recognition of the role of the nurse as a health educator and its implementation. Suominen (1993) assessed the extent to which breast cancer patients' information needs are met and found that nurses' perceptions of their health education role are unclear. In some cases, nurses believed information giving to be a 'medical issue' and therefore the responsibility of the doctor. This lack of clarity of the nurse's health education role was confirmed in a further study among a similar group of patients by Suominen *et al.* (1994).

The need for nurses to adopt a holistic approach to patients as individuals, supporting their active participation in a close and equal partnership and enabling the process of self-care through responsible health behaviour, was also identified by Kyngas and Hentinen (1995). This need was found to be fulfilled by nurses who perceived themselves to be empowered (Raatikainen, 1994). In her study, these empowered nurses were more often found to hold senior positions (nurse specialists or assistant head nurses), rather than to be working as 'registered nurses'. It was concluded that a more advanced level of nursing education, continuous professional development, the possession of a wider sense of responsibility, clearer principles and the ability to work in collaboration with others were the distinguishing features of an 'empowered' nurse. However, the study did not make clear whether or not these senior nurses were attempting, or were sufficiently empowered within the hierarchies of the five hospitals surveyed, to create supportive working environments for their junior nursing colleagues, which would in turn be empowering.

'Self-care' health educational programmes in Finland are predominantly based on counselling during individual patient contacts, by both registered nurses and public health nurses, in the hospitals and municipal health centres respectively. These programmes have been criticized for their tendency to rely on the application of a 'universal package', rather than being based on an appraisal of individual needs (Suominen, 1993; Miilunpalo *et al.*, 1995).

France

Historically, the role of nurses in France has been regulated by the content and omissions of several decrees. Since 1984, nurses have had the legal authority to assume a role in health education and health promotion but it was not until a decree in 1993 that nursing became an autonomous profession with its own explicit values and principles. Prior to this nurses were legally subordinate to a dominant medical profession by whom their work was prescribed, rather than being a complementary profession working in partnership. Lacroix (1992) described the struggle she experienced as the only nurse in France at that time to become President of a Departmental Committee for Health Education. She also emphasizes the considerable difficulties faced by nurses in gaining rightful recognition for the valuable contribution they can make as health educators as they remain under-represented and undervalued.

In 1992, a revised public health module, consistent with the principles of the Ottawa Charter for Health Promotion, was included in nursing education programmes leading to the

French State Diploma in Nursing. The goals of this module are to prepare nurses for multidisciplinary collaboration and their role as 'agents of health' and to enable them to participate effectively in the development of a real public health policy which, in the future, 'will have to be structured around a reflection on patient education that will drive him [the patient], little by little, to take some charge, by himself, of his illness' (Alozy, 1993, p. 29).

During this decade, there has been much discussion about nursing ethics and the autonomy of the patient in France. In relation to the role of the nurse as a health educator, there appears to be more of an expression of the right sentiments that endorse the self-empowerment of patients than practical strategies for overcoming some of the very real obstacles that separate nurses and patients. As in Finland and the United Kingdom, there is little written about the effect that the lack of autonomy has on the nurse's role as a health educator. Despite legal recognition of such a role and an education which provides an appropriate knowledge base, as well as teaching and communication skills which should, in theory, give nurses the necessary competence and confidence, external barriers to the performance of the role still exist. For example, Posko (1993), in a small survey of cancer patients' satisfaction with the information they were given, found that part of the problem in providing patients with the information they wanted was caused by insufficient communication between medical and nursing personnel. From the author's experience, the public hospital sector is generally understaffed by *infirmières* (first-level nurses) who, in their highly skilled, extended roles, are bound by an inflexible task-oriented organization.

Within such a system patients are denied the individualized assessment and care which is at the core of the new nursing philosophy, although when working with empowered patients and clients, nurses welcome the opportunity to encourage an active partnership. However, in a society that is conscious of consumerism, the self-employed community nurses (*infirmières soins à domicile* and *infirmières libérales*) may not always take opportunistic health education initiatives in relation to smoking, sensible drinking or practising safer sex, for fear of offending and losing a client and consequently reducing their income.

The exception may be when clients have a chronic disease or long-term disability and their partnership in care has become 'bonded'. In their role as health educators then, community nurses seem to represent a vast, relatively inexpensive (reimbursable), accessible, but greatly underutilized and under-recognized resource, both by the public, the policy-makers and the professionals themselves.

The United Kingdom

Some of the above comments may strike a common chord with the experiences of nurses working as health educators in the United Kingdom. Health education has been a well-established element in the role of community nurses and still comprises a large part of their health promotion work (Sourtzi *et al.*, 1996). These authors found that health education was largely based on traditional one-to-one activities. In the UK, the term 'community nurses' refers to practice nurses, health visitors, midwives, district nurses, school nurses, community psychiatric nurses, community mental handicap nurses, indeed any nurse working in primary health care settings.

Although the United Kingdom's 'Health of the Nation' strategy (Department of Health, 1992) recognizes the role of nurses in health education and health promotion, the recognition is a somewhat limited vision of what the role could be. For instance, one implication of this strategy in practice, through its targeting of high-risk groups and inadequate recognition of the socio-economic determinants of health, is the expectation that nurses will adopt a behaviour change approach. The strategy is not sufficiently supportive of the nurses' role as a facilitator of health education whose goal it is to empower patients and clients. Many opportunities are lost through, for example, statutory duties, case load size, collecting information on patients' health status and health surveillance, in fulfilment of the Health of the Nation targets.

Although in the United Kingdom hospital nurses exist in vast numbers, have close and continuous contact with patients and are knowledgeable about health education, Delaney (1994, p. 833), referring to two unpublished studies (Richardson, 1992;

Glossop, 1993), concludes that 'there is little evidence that it [health promotion] is rigorously and readily related to everyday practice' and this may also apply to health education. In hospital settings this is partly due to nurses' socialization into traditional practices such as ward organization and the expectations of colleagues, as well as the demands of the bureaucratic and hierarchical system in which they are employed.

Educating patients for health and self-care is seen as a priority in the recently reformed nursing education at Diploma level, commonly referred to as Project 2000 (Noble, 1991). These courses encompass holistic views of health, but as Delaney (1994) observes, a theory–practice gap is evident due to the lack of attention given to how abstract conceptual issues, such as enablement and empowerment, can be translated into the actual behavioural skills of the nurse.

Trnobranski (1994, p. 735) commented that a 'nurse needs to be empowered and have the freedom to make decisions as an autonomous practitioner, in order to be an agent of the patient's freedom of choice'. Nurses should be accountable for any professional decisions that they make. The UKCC in its *Code of Professional Conduct* (1992) expects practitioners to possess these attributes of autonomy and accountability. The extent of their realization within nursing in general, as well as in the 'facilitator' role of the nurse as health educator, is still, however, debatable (Trnobranski, 1994).

Conclusion

In Finland, France and the United Kingdom, the overall health of these populations has improved in recent years, for as people are more articulate and socially and economically advantaged, they tend to adopt healthier lifestyles. The goals of the Health For All 2000 strategy and its more radical Ottawa Charter for Health Promotion identify the need to reduce or eliminate differences between socio-economic groups and overcome health-damaging lifestyles. Throughout Europe, however, there remains a considerable problem aggravated by the economic recession of the 1990s.

The approach towards better health and the social and economic fulfilment of patients and clients through self-empowerment provides considerable challenges for nurses in their role as health educators. This, not surprisingly, may seem a daunting task for any individual or group of nurses although the process of achieving autonomy of the patient or client must have a beginning.

Based on the available literature, the extent to which nurses in all three countries are able to practise their role as health educators and perform it in an ethical manner is impossible to assess as further evaluative research is required. Existing evidence, however, indicates that lack of knowledge, patient assessment and communication skills, confidence and support from those who control their activities and employment may reduce the likelihood of effective health education if it is practised at all.

Disparities exist in all three countries between the aspirations of facilitating patients and clients towards the goal of self-empowerment and the realities of existing health education practices. These practices are more likely to exist somewhere along a continuum between the roles of expert practising activities within a behavioural change approach and that of facilitator whose approach is client-centred. Neither role is right or wrong in itself, but should be determined by the needs and wishes of the patients and clients involved, and realistically take into account the social, economic and political factors that influence their everyday lives.

The issues involved in respecting and promoting patient or client autonomy are closely related to and concern the degree of autonomy which nurses themselves possess. If health education is to be an ethical enterprise, there is a clear need, not only to empower patients and clients, but also to empower nurses in their role as health educators.

Acknowledgements

I would like to thank Win Tadd for her helpful comments and contribution to the discussion of the concept of health on pages 62–4.

References

Alozy, M. (1993) 'Une expérience de formation des élèves-infirmière en éducation pour la santé', *Soins Formation-Pédagogie-Encadrement*, **8**: 23–9.

Antrobus, S. (1997) 'An analysis of nursing in context: the effects of current health policy', *Journal of Advanced Nursing*, **25**: 447–53.

Bunton, R. and Macdonald, G. (1992) *Health Promotion: Disciplines and Diversity*. (Routledge: London).

Davis, S.M. (1995) 'An investigation into nurses' understanding of health education and health promotion within a neuro-rehabilitation setting', *Journal of Advanced Nursing*, **21**: 952–9.

Delaney, F.G. (1994) 'Nursing and health promotion: conceptual concerns', *Journal of Advanced Nursing*, **20**: 828–35.

Demeulemeester, R. and Baudier, F. (1995) 'Health promotion and education in France, a case-study', *Promotion and Education*, **II**: 22–35.

Department of Health (1992) *The Health of the Nation – A Strategy for Health in England*. (HMSO: London).

Eskola, J. (1995) 'Health promotion and education in Finland: a case study', *Promotion and Education*, **II**: 55–8.

Ewles, L. and Simnett, I. (1992) *Promoting Health: A Practical Guide*, 2nd edn. (Scutari Press: London).

Gallie, W.B. (1955–56) 'Essentially contested concepts', *Proceedings of the Aristotelian Society*, **56**: 167–98.

Glossop, D. (1993) 'Health education and health promotion', unpublished MSc dissertation, Leeds Metropolitan University, Leeds.

Hagard, S. (1995) 'Health promotion and education in England: a case study', *Promotion and Education*, **II**: 45–52.

Jewell, S.E. (1994) 'Patient participation: what does it mean to nurses?', *Journal of Advanced Nursing*, **19**: 433–8.

Kyngas, H. and Hentinen, M. (1995) 'Meaning attached to compliance with self-care, and conditions for compliance among young diabetics', *Journal of Advanced Nursing*, **21**: 729–36.

Lacroix, H. (1992) 'Infirmière et Presidente d'un Comite Departemental d'Education pour la santé', *Revue de l'Infirmière*, **14**: 48–50.

Lalonde, M. (1974) *A New Perspective on the Health of Canadians*. (Information Canada: Ottawa).

Latter, S., Macleod Clark, J., Wilson-Barnett, J. and Maben, J. (1992) 'Health education in nursing: perceptions of practice in acute settings', *Journal of Advanced Nursing*, **17**: 164–72.

Lindley, R. (1986) *Autonomy*. (Macmillan: London).

McBride, A. (1994) 'Health promotion in hospitals: the attitudes, beliefs and practices of hospital nurses', *Journal of Advanced Nursing*, **20**: 92–100.

Manicot, C. (1991) 'Médecine du travail, au coeur de l'usine', *Revue de l'Infirmière*, **1**: 18–26.

Marty, F. And Macaux, M. (1997) 'Chirurgie du sein: informer les patientes', *Objectif Soins*, **1**: 30–7.

May, C.M. (1995) 'Patient autonomy and the politics of professional relationships', *Journal of Advanced Nursing*, **21**: 83–7.

Miilunpalo, S., Laitakari, J. and Vuori, I. (1995) 'Strengths and weaknesses in health counselling in Finnish primary health care', *Patient Education and Counselling*, **2**: 317–28.

Noble, C. (1991) 'Are nurses good patient educators?', *Journal of Advanced Nursing*, **6**: 1185–9.

Nordenfelt, L. (1993) *Quality of Life, Health and Happiness*. (Avebury: Aldershot).

Posko, C. (1993) 'Prise en charge de malades cancereux', *Soins*, **575/6**: 63–71.

Raatikainen, R. (1994) 'Power or lack of it in nursing care', *Journal of Advanced Nursing*, **19**: 424–32.

Richardson, K. (1992) 'The perceived health promotion role of hospital-based nurses in Trafford: a qualitative study into practices and problems, unpublished MSc dissertation, Leeds Polytechic, Leeds.

Salvage, J. (1990) 'Theory and practice of the 'new nursing', occasional paper, *Nursing Times*, **86**: 42–5.

Siivola, U. and Martikainen, T. (1990) 'The public health nurse – the linchpin of primary health care', *World Health Forum*, **11**: 102–7.

Sourtzi, P., Nolan, P. and Andrews, R. (1996) 'Evaluation of health promotion activities in community nursing practice', *Journal of Advanced Nursing*, **24**: 1214–23.

Suominen, T. (1993) 'How do nurses assess the information received by breast cancer patients?', *Journal of Advanced Nursing*, **18**: 64–8.

Suominen, T., Leino-Kilpi, H. and Laippala, P. (1994) 'Nurses' role in informing breast cancer patients: a comparison between patients' and nurses' opinions', *Journal of Advanced Nursing*, **19**: 6–11.

Tadd, W. (1995) 'Moral agency and the role of the nurse', unpublished PhD thesis, University of Wales, Cardiff.

Tessier, S., Andreys, J-B. and Ribiero, M-A. (1996) *Santé Publique et Santé Communautaire*. (Maloine: Paris).

Trnobranski, P. H. (1994) 'Nurse–patient negotiation: assumption or reality?', *Journal of Advanced Nursing*, **19**: 733–7.

United Kingdom Central Council for Nursing, Midwifery and Health Visiting (1992) *Code of Professional Conduct*, 3rd edn. *Nursing*, **22**: 731–7.

Vehviläinen-Julkunen, K. (1992) 'Client–public health nurse relationships in child health care: a grounded theory study', *Journal of Advanced Nursing*, **17**: 896–904.

Vehviläinen-Julkunen, K. (1995) 'Family training: supporting mothers and fathers in the transition to parenthood', *Journal of Advanced Nursing*, **22**: 731–7.

Waterworth, S. and Luker, K. (1990) 'Reluctant collaborators: do patients want to be involved in decisions concerning care?' *Journal of Advanced Nursing*, **15**: 971–6.

World Health Organization (1948) *Constitution*. (WHO: Geneva).

World Health Organization (1978) *Report on the International Conference on Primary Health Care*, Alma Ata, 6–12 September. (WHO: Geneva).

World Health Organization (1984) 'Health promotion: A discussion document on the concept and principles', WHO Regional Office for Europe: Copenhagen, reprinted in *Health Promotion*, **1**(1): 73–6.

World Health Organization (1985) *Targets for Health for All*. (WHO: Copenhagen).

World Health Organization (1986) *Ottawa Charter for Health Promotion. An International Conference on Health Promotion*, Ottawa, Canada, 17–21 November (WHO: Copenhagen).

Suggestions for further reading

Bunton, R. and Macdonald, G. (1992) *Health Promotion: Disciplines and Diversity*. (Routledge: London).

Doxiadis, S. (1990) *Ethics in Health Education*. (John Wiley & Sons: Chichester).

Ewles, L. and Simnett, I. (1992) *Promoting Health: A Practical Guide*, 2nd edn. (Scutari Press: London).

Kiger, A.M. (1995) *Teaching for Health*, 2nd edn. (Churchill Livingstone: Edinburgh).

Naidoo, J. and Wills, J. (1944) *Health Promotion: Foundations for Practice*. (Baillière Tindall: London).

Nordenfelt, L. (1993) *Quality of Life, Health and Happiness*. (Avebury: Aldershot).

Scriven, A. and Orme, J. (1996) *Health Promotion: Professional Perspectives*. (The Open University Press: London).

Seedhouse, D. (1988) *Ethics: The Heart of Health Care*. (John Wiley & Sons: Chichester).

Sidell, M., Jones, L., Katz, J. and Peberdy, A. (eds) (1997) *Debates and Dilemmas in Promoting Health: A Reader*. (Macmillan: Basingstoke).

5

Community Nursing: The Ethical Issues

Rosie Tope and June Smail

Introduction

During recent years many of the countries forming the continent of Europe have become more closely integrated in terms of health and social policy. Inevitably this integration of policy has influenced the mode of management, organization and delivery of patient care. Most European countries have adopted the WHO philosophy of 'Health for All by the Year 2000' and have been working with varying degrees of success towards achieving this aim. In 1993, the Council of Europe concluded that the adoption of a common strategy in the fields of public health and welfare would achieve a greater unity between its members. The adoption of this strategy enabled professionals involved in health and social care to train and work throughout Europe in the country of their choice.

Most countries now boast pluralistic societies in which a diversity of people live. Many different ethnic, racial, religious and social groups can be identified, all of whom wish to maintain independent lifestyles and retain their own values while living within a common civilization. Recognition of and respect for the rights and views of others enhance the quality of health and social care. Ethnocentricity has no place in society if Health for All is to remain an achievable target.

As a result of the 1993 Council of Europe recommendations, most European countries are formally adopting the concept of collaboration in health and social care on both national and international bases. Furthermore, a great emphasis is placed on the contribution made by effective teamworking. The White Paper *Caring for People* (DoH, 1990) laid out plans for 'community care in the next decade and beyond'. The main aims were identified as promoting individual choice and independence by:

- Enabling people to live as normal a life as possible in their own homes or in a homely environment in the local community
- Providing the right amount of care and support to help people achieve maximum possible independence.

The primary health care team (PHCT) has a vital role to play in helping the general population to achieve these aims. General practices are the focus of community provision and there are clear implications for teamworking as a mechanism for co-ordinating community care.

Structure and organization of primary health care in Europe

The core members of primary health care teams vary considerably throughout Europe. In many countries registered nurses work solely within the primary health care centres and do not visit patients in their homes. Instead, patients are expected to visit the health centres for consultation and treatment. Most countries do not have the equivalent qualification of health visitor and most tend to use the generic term 'community nurse'. In addition, many of the primary health centres fulfil the function of a small hospital by providing in-patient beds. In some countries the health centres are the first port of call for all emergency and urgent care, rather than the model adopted in the UK of accident and emergency departments located in district general hospitals.

Within the confines of this chapter, it is not feasible to examine the organization and delivery of community care in every country in Europe, but opinions have been sought from experts in primary health care in Greece, Finland and Sweden. These individuals have considered the ethical dilemmas commonly faced by nurses and the other professionals working in the community within their own countries. In our analysis of their comments it will be seen that common beliefs and aspirations emerge, along with a recognition of the effects of current circumstances and limitations within which all primary health care teams currently function.

Each of the countries discussed supports the notion that it is preferable for people to be cared for in their own homes wherever possible and that the core value of health care should be the worth, dignity and individuality of every patient. There are similar concerns about the cost of institutionalized care and the need to secure adequate funding for chronically ill and elderly people. Most of all, there is concern about the seeming inability of the various organizations and authorities to work collaboratively and harmoniously for the good of the patient. There is a similar recognition that acute sector care has always attracted, and for the foreseeable future will continue to attract, the greatest amount of financial investment. There is great concern that these apparently insurmountable problems will continue to impede progress in enhancing the quality of community care.

Political, historical and cultural influences all play a part in the philosophical interpretation which each country applies to its planning and implementation of health care and it is these differences upon which this chapter focuses. Therefore, before considering the most prevalent ethical issues, the structure and organization of primary health care within the four selected countries will be described.

Ethical issues concerning professional accountability, autonomy, advocacy, clinical judgement and competence are considered in conjunction with the rights and expectations of patients regarding confidentiality, informed consent, compliance and invasion of privacy. A central tenet of the discussion is that ethics is not just a matter of personal opinion, and therefore any decision reached about a particular ethical issue is bound to raise some controversy.

When caring for patients in the community, nurses and health visitors are confronted by many conflicting needs and interests. For example, the prevailing social factors may not only conflict with the existing economic and political limitations, but also test the personal integrity of individual practitioners. The difficulties for practitioners lie in justifying what is right and good and in using their insights gained from systematic, reflective study to influence the development of ethical health policies.

How the ethical issues are addressed has been analysed and described by community health professionals in Greece, Sweden and Finland, so that the similarities and differences can be highlighted and compared with UK practice.

The United Kingdom

In the UK the roles of all nurses working in community settings have evolved rapidly over the last few years. Frequently, they are based in the same premises as, and work in collaboration with, general practitioners as core members of the primary health care team. In 1996, the Department of Health indicated that there were 8999 general practices and health centres in England and 532 in Wales (DoH, 1996a).

A primary health care team is generally accepted as being an association of different professionals whose aim is to provide the patient with comprehensive care (RCGP, 1991). The roles of individual team members may vary, but the purposes and goals of the team should be clear and shared. Effective care delivery requires that nurses and health visitors co-ordinate and plan care with the involvement of clients, patients and other professionals.

In the UK, health visitors provide a service to families, especially those with young children, across all social classes and age groups. The four guiding principles of health visiting which remain relevant today are:

- The search for health needs
- The stimulation of awareness of health needs
- The influence of policies affecting health
- The facilitation of health-enhancing activities (CETHV, 1977).

Community nurses work predominantly in people's homes, with the elderly, those who are chronically sick or those who are terminally ill. Many of their patients, therefore, are those whose problems 'defy precise definition, do not have readily available cures and are often prolonged' (Knopke and Diekelman, 1981). Although community nurses work as independent practitioners, they are managerially accountable to nurse managers and are usually employees of an NHS trust.

In the main, practice nurses are employed by general practitioners (GPs) and work in health centres and GP surgeries. In recent years, their numbers have increased dramatically in response to the 1990 GP contract. This new contract, imposed on GPs by the government, not only includes a number of new controls on GP activities, but also extended the services which GPs are expected provide to include more health promotion and illness prevention. Practice nurses represent approximately 20 per cent of all nurses working in primary care (Atkin and Lunt, 1993) and their role includes investigative procedures, screening and health promotion activities, family planning, chronic disease management, childhood immunization, travel health and advising on minor ailments.

These three groups of community nurses, health visitors, district nurses and practice nurses, make up the 'core' nursing component of primary health care teams. In addition community midwives, community psychiatric nurses and school nurses increasingly work as team members in GP practices. Midwives are responsible for the total care of women during pregnancy and the postnatal period. The community psychiatric nurse's skills are particularly helpful to people who have depression, mental stress and/or dementia and school nurses liaise with the practice, schools and families on child health issues.

When the organization of community nurses in the UK is compared with that of other European countries, different patterns emerge.

Greece

Greece has been trying to implement a national health service for the past 15 years, with varying degrees of success. The latest reform occurred in 1992 when Greece was divided into a number of district health services. The geographical size and patient population of each district vary considerably, depending on whether it is in an urban or rural location. Each district health service has a director who represents its interests at the Central Health Committee which is directly answerable to the Ministry of Health. According to Greek law (Law No. 2071), the Greek state secures the right of every citizen to seek and gain access to primary, secondary and tertiary health care, while at the same time enabling each individual to retain freedom of choice and dignity. The Central Health Committee comprises several doctors representing the clinical sector, a doctor and dentist who represent the university medical and dental schools respectively, a representative (usually a doctor) from the schools of nursing, one senior nurse who represents all the secondary and tertiary care nurses of Greece and finally the Director of Social Services.

Primary health care for 10 million people is provided by 185 health centres situated throughout Greece. Each health centre serves at least four communities and has at least four peripheral clinics. The centres develop their own policies which reflect the needs of their respective populations (National Statistical Office of Greece, 1993). Halandritsa health centre, situated 22 kilometres from Patras, for example, was opened in its present form in 1991. It serves 27 villages located over a wide geographical area with a total population of 25,000 people. Five peripheral clinics are run by the staff from the health centre which is autonomous.

Organizational policy is developed by the core team consisting of the medical director, other doctors, nurses, midwives, social workers and administrative staff. The health centre is managed and organized by an innovative, enthusiastic and committed medical director and staff and as such, serves as an exemplar for many other health centres. Great emphasis is placed on health education and health promotion for all patients, as well as the provision of innovative in-service continuing education programmes for trained staff and students from a number of professions. The health centre acts as the focal point for the population. Social activities take place within the centre with people from many different villages attending. There is an integral link between many of the health and social activities and a clear health education message. Lack of resources, however, impedes further developments which the Halandritsa team are keen to implement.

In some areas of Greece, additional primary health care may be provided by out-patient clinics in the district hospitals providing this is approved by the hospital council. Efstathiou (1997) suggests that after almost 15 years of an established primary health service in Greece, the following general conclusions can be drawn:

- Curative services are still in high demand
- There is no national strategy regarding primary health care
- There is a great shortage of qualified nursing staff and social workers
- There is a chronic lack of resources which impede progress in primary health care
- Many of the professions retain a traditional orientation towards curative rather than preventative care.

Finland

The central tenet of Finland's health policy is to 'encourage people to adopt healthier ways of living, reduce preventable health problems, and refine and elaborate the health service network' (Ministry of Social Affairs and Health [MSAH], 1996, p. 5). Priority has been given to the community sector and the organization and delivery of health care have been modified accordingly. Staff who originally worked in acute hospital settings are being transferred to newly created posts in the community. All patients with non-urgent problems are assessed by a medical practitioner within three working days and, if necessary, are referred to a hospital for further investigation within one or two weeks of the initial consultation.

Finland's health policy has meant that 'the health of the population has steadily improved even though disparities between sectors of the population still exist' (MSAH, 1996, p. 1). Generally, however, people have adopted healthier lifestyles in recent years, although there tends to be a higher number of deaths through accidents, suicides and acts of violence in Finland than in most other European countries. Conversely, the number of deaths from cancer tends to be lower although the reasons for this are not clear.

In 1994 there were 243 health centres in 455 municipalities serving a total population of just over 5 million people. In order to ensure continuity of care, the local populations served by the health centres are organized into 'cells' of between 4000 and 10,000 people. Each cell is assigned to a team which comprises doctors, public health nurses and other professionals. Each doctor has responsibility for approximately 2000 patients. The system is comparable with that in the United Kingdom as each patient registers with an individual general practitioner in a health centre. In normal circumstances, the patient makes an appointment to see his or her own doctor, but anyone requesting an urgent referral is able to see the first doctor available.

The total number of in-patient beds in the health centres is 23,000 or 451 beds per 100,000 inhabitants and only 13 centres are without in-patient beds. Arrangements for home visits by community nurses are the responsibility of the health centres and the majority of these visits are to patients over 65 years of age.

Sweden

Sweden has a population of almost 9 million people, with 85 per cent living in the southern half of the country (Svenska Institutet, 1994). Health and social care are viewed as crucial to the overall welfare of the country and both are financed through a national social insurance system. There are 10 regional hospitals, 80 district or county hospitals and 900 health centres serving the entire population and approximately 300,000 people are employed in the health care sector (Svenska Institutet, 1995). In general, Sweden's population enjoys a relatively high standard of health when compared with international standards. Life expectancy is rising with 18 per cent of the population over 65 years of age and infant mortality is one of the lowest in the world. Cardiovascular diseases account for more than half of all deaths. In common with other Scandinavian countries the incidence of suicide is relatively high, although this has decreased significantly during the last decade. There are, however, considerable and growing differences in the level of health attained by different social groups (Svenska Institutet, 1995).

The primary health care centre is the first point of contact with the health service for the population. Individuals have the right to choose their own family doctor who treats all diseases and injuries not requiring hospital admission. Many different health professionals are employed by the health centres. All patients pay a fee for each consultation and this has recently been increased to 125Kr which is approximately £12.50. After a total fee of 800Kr is paid in any one year any additional consultations are free. In 1997, however, there is emerging evidence that people cannot afford to seek treatment and care and it is anticipated that the gap will widen still further between the different levels of health experienced by the different social classes. In addition, there are a number of private schemes available and many people consult a doctor and receive treatment through this route.

Patients do not have access to health centres 24 hours a day. If someone is ill during the night or at weekends the district hospital is contacted for advice. An established community nursing service provides home visits when required and a number of clinics within the health centres are nurse or midwife led.

In a pattern reminiscent of other Western countries, the largest proportion of financial resources, 58 per cent, is allocated to the acute care sector with only 5 per cent being spent on long-term care and 17 per cent on primary health care. In total 7.5 per cent of the gross national product is spent on health care (Svenska Institutet, 1995).

In 1992, as a result of lengthening waiting lists, a guarantee was introduced that no patient should wait more than three months for admission to hospital. If the patient's local hospital is unable to meet this criterion, then arrangements must be made to admit the patient to an alternative hospital. During the same period, the number of beds in acute, psychiatric and long-term care facilities has reduced considerably with the introduction of policies to enable individuals to remain in their own homes wherever feasible. It is reported that many patients have been discharged from hospital into the community without appropriate support or funding and, in common with the United Kingdom, this has caused an additional strain on the under-funded primary health care sector.

Ethical issues

Policy development and allocation of resources

In a truly pluralistic society, effective community care raises a number of ethical issues. Questions about what constitutes a priority are being increasingly debated by health and social service personnel in the UK, Greece, Finland and Sweden, as well as in numerous other countries. Strategic planners, policy-makers and managers may differ significantly in their percep-tions of need from those of clinical staff who are at the sharp end of patient or client care. Although limited financial resources are still widely perceived as the most crucial limiting factor in primary health care, issues of quality and safety are increasingly entering the equation. Ways are being sought to ensure that the same priority is given to caring for chroni-cally sick and elderly people in the final stages of their lives, as to those with acute illnesses or injuries who require life-saving treatment.

There is a significant cultural difference between some of the southern and northern European countries as far as caring for frail elderly people is concerned. In northern Europe the nuclear family is in much greater evidence, while in southern Europe it is commonplace for three or even four generations of a family to live together. There it is usual for younger family members to care for frail, elderly relatives in the family home. There is, therefore, less demand on both health and social service sectors to care for and financially support elderly people. Although this may be of great psychological benefit to the elderly person concerned, it may also disadvantage them as there is less opportunity for health professionals to assess and treat their physical needs. Caring for a dependent relative on a 24-hour basis also places a heavy burden on the carers. In Greece, for example, many women forgo the opportunity to pursue a career because it is expected that they will care for all their dependent relatives. This burden is compounded even more by the lack of qualified community nurses able to visit patients in their own homes.

Balancing interests

Many ethical issues can be attributed to the need to balance the rights and quality of life of an individual against the need to use limited resources appropriately. This means that patients wishing to exercise their autonomy in relation to treatment decisions may not be able to because of a lack of resources. Dines and Cribb (1993) argued that autonomy is an integral part of human health and well-being. In some instances, however, the health and autonomy of an individual may conflict with the health and economic well-being of the community in which he or she lives.

Downie and Calman (1987) queried what restrictions, if any, should be placed on individuals who represent a potential danger to the health of the community in which they live. Furthermore, they asked whether infringing the liberty of an individual in order to improve the health of others can ever be justified. In some instances the answer would appear to be quite clear. In the United Kingdom, a person who is deemed to be severely mentally ill and is thought to be a danger, either to himself or to others, can be compulsorily detained in a secure place. An individual who is known to have salmonella and who handles food intended for consumption by the general public will be forbidden to work on health grounds, until he is clear of the infection. People who refuse to practise safe sex while knowing that they are HIV positive have been identified publicly. Similarly, in Scandinavia strict controls are placed on individuals representing a danger to the public. In Sweden, for example, an individual who is HIV positive is required by law to give the names of any sexual partners and to inform them that they are carrying the virus.

In Greece the situation is less clear. As far as the person with salmonella and working in the food industry is concerned, the law forbids that person to work until the infection is cleared.

The problem, and therefore the ethical dilemma, is that employers may not enforce this even if they are aware of the situation. The only people who may be aware that a person has salmonella are the health professionals and, if they protect patient confidentiality, they put members of the general public at risk. In reality, it is left to the patient to decide. The question of identifying individuals who are HIV positive but who do not practise safe sex is a subject of current debate in Greece. As yet no conclusions have been drawn.

In other instances the situation may be more confused, for example parents refusing to have their children immunized or women refusing cervical smears or mammograms and wishing to be removed from call and recall programmes. It could, for instance, be argued that as patients or clients have the right to agree to or refuse treatment, a health professional is accountable only for ensuring that the person is in possession of all the facts to enable informed decision-making which reflects personal choice and preferences. In Greece, parents who refuse to have their children immunized are prosecuted. Parents are legally responsible for their children's health until they reach 18 years of age. This is similar to Finland, where 'a child's parent is not entitled to refuse treatment that would avert a health risk or save the life of a minor' (MSAH, 1996, p. 8). With regard to personal choice, however, a woman can refuse to have a cervical smear or a mammogram as she is not deemed to place anyone but herself at risk.

Seedhouse and Lovett (1992) argued that clinical and ethical analysis and decision-making are inseparable in health care. They suggested that clinical analysis entails identifying the patient's or client's problem, making the correct diagnosis, deciding the appropriate treatment and determining how the treatment should be organized and managed. Ethical analysis, on the other hand, involves the identification of the role and duties of the health professional in clinical analysis, what the preferred outcome should be for the client and how much time a health professional should devote to achieving that preferred outcome. A further critical consideration is the extent to which a patient's or client's ability to be self-governing should be respected. This decision must be made in conjunction with deliberations about how much information should be given and how authoritative a health professional should be.

While there appears to be little doubt that clinical and ethical analysis are inseparable, it is the interpretation and application of the latter which presents the major challenge in primary health care. Professional ethics and the ethics of daily living are not radically different and it is argued that the ethical issues which arise within the confines of community care cannot be minimized through devising clinical protocols.

Patients' rights

In Europe there appears to be a general consensus of opinion regarding the overall clinical diagnosis, treatment and management of patients, but here the similarity ends. The way in which patient and client care is organized and delivered, how much information is given and the degree of patient participation in care differ significantly between the various countries. To a large extent these differences depend on the historical development, policy decisions and the ethnic, racial and cultural influences which have evolved in the individual countries. Since the beginning of this decade a number of countries have introduced Patient Charters (DoH, 1996b) or Bills of Rights. In essence many of these documents say the same thing. For instance, a patient must consent to treatment and should do so after a full explanation of their state of health. The diagnosis, the extent of treatment and care needed, the risk factors involved and any feasible alternatives to the recommended course of action should form part of any such explanations if they are to qualify as ethical and demonstrate respect for the individuals concerned.

In Greece, however, no such Bill of Rights exists. Although many patients in Greece may be aware of their diagnosis, it is by no means certain that everyone asks or is told the nature of their illness or the expected outcome. This is particularly true if a person has cancer. Culturally, people tend to avoid using the word 'cancer' and several authors suggest that cancer is still regarded as a stigma. Many Greeks refer to cancer as 'the bad disease'. All patients are given the opportunity of being informed of their diagnoses but many prefer being kept in ignorance. Patients also have the right to refuse recommended treatments and, in common with most other countries, are then held responsible for the consequences. Community nurses are seen as having an essential role in helping patients recognize and understand the treatment they are receiving.

In all four countries patients are entitled to read their personal health records and, with the exception of Greece, are able to amend any information they believe to be inaccurate. Complaints procedures are explicit and personal health records are deemed to be confidential with access only allowed to those capable of justifying it. In Greece, patients and their relatives are given the relevant information by the doctor. No other health professional is allowed to disclose new information. For community nurses this can prove difficult, as they are not permitted to answer any additional questions asked by patients. On discharge from hospital, most patients receive information pamphlets which are then used by community nurses as a basis for discussion with their clients.

In the UK, professional accountability requires that community nurses have the authority to act with a reasonable degree of autonomy. There are, of course, areas of potential conflict with fellow nurses, other professionals and managerial personnel. The attributes of accountability and autonomy are authorized within the nurses' *Code of Professional Conduct* (UKCC, 1992). In Finland and Sweden, community nurses are also held accountable for their practice. Nurses in Greece, however, do not work independently from the doctor, whether in a patient's home or the health centre, thus their accountability is to the doctor rather than to the patient. It is, for example, a nurse's professional duty to inform the doctor of any confidential information pertaining to the patient's health problem, regardless of how or where this is obtained.

Justice and inequalities

For many community nurses in the United Kingdom, the re-organization of the health service in 1990 and the introduction of the GP contract have raised ethical concerns in relation to equity. Fund-holding general practitioners carry their own budgets to purchase patient care and this has been criticized for encouraging a two-tier system which benefits these patients to the detriment of others (Harmen, 1996). Similarly, the allocation of scarce resources within a market economy is currently of ethical concern to many community nurses.

It has already been acknowledged by the Svenska Institutet that there is a growing concern in Sweden about the widening gap in the level of health attained by different social classes. Failure to provide adequate financial support for primary health care can only increase the health risks to poorer members of society. This in turn places greater financial demands on the acute care sector which then has to respond to the increasing need for secondary or tertiary treatment and care.

In Finland, exactly the same trends are identified. Fund-holding is a municipal responsibility and currently there are real concerns concerning the equitable distribution of some budgets and resources allocated to the primary health centres. In 1997, the Ministry of Social Affairs and Health itself acknowledged that the health service in general has been subject to major cuts in the money available as well as to inequitable distribution of existing funds. Since 1991, the number of staff employed in health and social care has decreased significantly. There are 46,000 professionals working in the primary health care sector in Finland but there are a further 31,000 doctors, nurses and social workers who are not employed because of a lack of funding. It has been suggested that if many of the unemployed health professionals were given jobs in primary health care, the country would save money in two ways. First, unemployment payments would be reduced and second, the level of health within the general population would improve as a result of more efficient primary health services.

The Ministry of Social Affairs and Health acknowledges, in the same document, that while the policy of reducing institutionalized care and decreasing the number of acute beds has been implemented successfully, there are inadequacies in the present system of care and support for people in the community. The number of psychiatric in-patient beds has been reduced by 35 per cent in five years. The additional demand for the services of the primary health care teams, by those patients unable to care adequately for themselves, is a cause of great concern and debate among community nurses.

At the beginning of 1997, a new law was enacted which determines minimum standards of care which must be achieved in private nursing homes. In a move similar to that which exists in the UK, nursing home inspectors with statutory powers to recommend closure of nursing homes which do not meet minimum standards have been appointed. Each municipality will be able to withdraw or withhold funding for unsatisfactory nursing homes. There is, however, general agreement that standards in most nursing homes are excellent and that compulsory closure will rarely need to be enforced.

In the UK, community services are criticized for being 'service driven' rather than 'needs led', but services based on need are often difficult to realize. Increasingly, health and social services are working in isolation instead of forming new alliances. Different services, such as needs assessment, treatment and care services, have to be co-ordinated to ensure that all of a patient's or client's needs are met.

In each primary health centre in Finland, the management team, which comprises a senior doctor, senior nurse and administrator, decides how their designated budget is to be allocated. The financial plans are then submitted for approval to a politically appointed council of lay people who approve or reject the proposals. A potential area of criticism is that as the council consists of political appointees, decisions on spending reflect the current political agenda rather than patient or client need. This again can cause major ethical dilemmas for the whole management team, as the need to seek approval may outweigh existing clinical priorities.

Interprofessional working

In the context of the health care team, conflicts and disagreements can arise between nurses and doctors as to who has ultimate authority and control over patient care (Tope, 1996). Thompson *et al.* (1988) suggested that although nurses may be left with the responsibility for patients they have no authority to change doctors' orders. Co-operation in planning patient care in a practice is essential. Protocols, when they are developed, agreed and used by both nurses and doctors, overcome possible conflicts about care and treatment. Protocols are used increasingly in the UK, Finland, Sweden and Greece and it is generally agreed that they help team members to collaborate more fully in planning and implementing patient care and treatment.

Another potential problem in relation to teamworking is confidentiality. Virtually all general practices in the UK use computers which can be programmed to allow differential access to the various team members. But how much patient confidence should be shared with other team members in order to manage a situation effectively? Decisions about disclosure of potentially confidential information must, by necessity, be a matter of professional judgement. The UKCC (1996, p. 26) states that 'confidentiality should only be broken in exceptional circumstances and should only occur after careful consideration that you can justify your action'.

In Finland, the Patient's Bill of Rights 1991 states quite clearly that under no circumstances can any information given by the patient, in confidence to a nurse or any other health professional, be disclosed. Unlike the UKCC directive, there is no written caveat that states 'in exceptional circumstances' confidential information can be shared on a 'need to know' basis. This presents a major ethical dilemma for Finnish community nurses as it is acknowledged that there are occasions when failure to disclose information may place the patient, or others, at risk. This is the complete antithesis of the Greek approach where all information must be disclosed to the doctor.

In Greece, the introduction of computers for record keeping is perceived to have benefited the entire health care team, as the previous medical secrecy has, to a large extent, been abolished. Nurses are no longer unaware of patients' health problems as the patient's records are available to anyone who has access to the computer. It remains, however, the responsibility of the nurse to maintain patient confidentiality from everyone other than the doctor. The number of health care teams evolving in Greece is increasing, in hospitals, clinics and health centres, and these are always managed and supervised by the doctor. The community nurse's prime responsibility in such teams is that of 'counsellor'.

Confidentiality and adolescents

In the UK, confidentiality relating to those aged under 16 is frequently concerned with issues surrounding family planning, drug and alcohol abuse, and at times these can pose particular ethical dilemmas for community nurses. The House of Lords decision in the Gillick case supported the view that in exceptional circumstances, treatment and medicine can be given to a girl under 16 years of age without the parents being informed (Dimond, 1990).

In Finland and Sweden there is no legal age of consent so that children of 12 are deemed to be capable of making an informed decision about their treatment and care. Theoretically, a girl of 12 could decide to have an abortion without informing her parents although, of course, this would be most unusual. Written consent forms are not common in many countries and therefore the dilemma of treating a child confidentially poses less of a problem for community nurses in Scandinavia than for those in the UK.

In Greece, parents have to be informed by law, if their daughter is less than 16 years of age and requests contraception. Doctors and nurses can offer advice and teaching about the various methods of contraception, but these cannot be prescribed without parental permission. Similarly, if a young person tells a health professional in confidence that they are using drugs, their parents must be informed of the situation by the health professional. From this standpoint there is no ethical dilemma for health professionals, as the law dictates that parents must be informed. The dilemma for community nurses and doctors is that because of the law, many young people do not seek appropriate advice and health care because they know that their parents will be informed. In order to meet the health needs of young people, some health professionals in Greece believe that the law should be more flexible.

Professional duties

Advocacy in health care is concerned with promoting and safeguarding the well-being and interests of patients and clients

(UKCC, 1996). Advocating for others may cause community nurses to compromise either themselves or their integrity as they attempt to uphold both the interests of service users and remain loyal to their employers. Examples of conflict may include complaints about low staffing levels or inappropriate skill mix. A particular problem for community nurses might be the early discharge of a patient from hospital in the absence of acceptable community care arrangements, which, in the UK, is now a social service responsibility. Increasingly, community nurses are taking the initiative and making their own decisions based on their own experience and education. *The Scope of Professional Practice* (UKCC, 1992) rejects the notion of 'role extension' and focuses instead on the autonomous practitioner. Nurses working in the community have expanded their practice and some have developed the nurse practitioner role. The Royal College of Nursing Institute of Advanced Nursing Education (RCNIANE, 1989) defines the nurse practitioner as someone who:

- Makes professional autonomous decisions, for which she/he has sole responsibility
- Possesses a repertoire of skills which embraces those with physical, psychological and social domains, especially diagnosing, prescribing, counselling and health promotion.

In Finland and Sweden, the term 'nurse practitioner' is not generally used, but there is clear evidence that community nurses in these countries fulfil the criteria necessary to claim this title. Experienced and expert nurses are permitted to make autonomous decisions, providing they are in full possession of the facts. Most of the skills and knowledge demonstrated by nurse practitioners in the UK are shared by their Scandinavian counterparts. However, in Finland, nurses are not permitted to prescribe drugs of any kind, neither are they supposed to give contraceptive advice. In reality, it seems that most will give informal advice at the request of a patient providing the circumstances are appropriate. In Greece, there is no current provision for the role of nurse practitioner, although there is no doubt that community nurses have a much more significant role than in previous decades.

Examples of the expanding role of the nurse can be seen in the mobile blood donation units which are organized and administered by experienced nurses.

Competence

Unless there is specific statutory legislation which requires a particular professional to carry out certain activities, there is considerable freedom for the development of skills which cross traditional lines of professional demarcation. The current emphasis in nursing is placed upon skills, knowledge and competence. However, Hunt and Wainwright (1994) ask, 'how do nurses know when they are competent, how does the employer determine the competence of an individual employee and how do the profession and the law courts determine competence?'

The problem of defining competence is one that appears to tax the nursing profession in each country under discussion. In common with the UK, the ethical issues surrounding incompetence are ones which are commonly debated in Finland, Sweden and Greece. All seem to agree that incompetence is evident on rare occasions, not only among the nursing profession but also within medicine and the professions allied to medicine. The problem it seems is not in identifying the incompetent practitioner, but is in the immediate 'closed door policy' which accompanies such an occurrence. In each country it is claimed that any investigation into incompetence is usually instigated as the result of a complaint by patients, or their relatives. Interviewing witnesses and collecting written evidence against an individual are fraught with difficulties because professional colleagues perceive their participation as disloyalty. In all four countries, there is a national Central Registration system. If a qualified nurse is removed from the Register, then theoretically, it should not be possible for him or her to gain employment as a qualified practitioner, although there is a suggestion that in Greece, some nurses work in private clinics after dismissal from the national health service. The general position in Greece, however, is that if a nurse does not perform his or her duties competently, the Administrative Council is informed and after due consideration, will decide the penalty that the nurse should pay.

Conclusion

In conclusion, the different approaches to ethical issues in the four countries described indicate the breadth of the area with which community nursing ethics is concerned. All community nurses and health visitors must practise their professions with due regard to the ethical principles which govern them, as well as in accordance with local policies, protocols and the law.

There can be no doubt that the 1990s is a period of enormous change in the organization and delivery of health care in the UK, Greece, Finland and Sweden. There has been a reduction in the length of hospital stays, a dramatic increase in the demand for community care and the boundaries, not only between health and social care, but also between the various professions involved, are being redrawn. There is also increased pressure to demonstrate consumer-orientated cost and clinically effective care within a competitive market.

The WHO regards the development of primary health care as one of the key elements in achieving 'Health for All' (WHO, 1995). The underlying principle is to provide an effective and efficient first-level contact for all families and individuals, near or in their own homes. However, the provision of care in the community is complex. There is a need for comprehensive liaison and collaboration between the hospital, community and social services for many age groups and conditions. Community nurses in all countries need to be aware of the influences of social, economical, political and ethical factors which may not be fully apparent in hospital. As the community health care setting has changed and continues to change, it is important that ethical concerns are identified and confronted in order to promote best practice and high-quality patient care.

Acknowledgements

The authors are indebted to the following people whose time, expertise and contribution have been invaluable in the writing of this chapter.

Dr Pangiotis Theodoropoulos; Dr Ioanna Theodoropoulou; Ms Sofia Kastana, Halandritsa Health Centre, Patras, Greece.

Ms Hilkka Sidoroff, Faculty of Health Sciences, North Karelia Polytechnic, Finland.
Dr Margareta Carlsson, College of Health Sciences, University of Boras, Sweden.
Ms Margareta Beierholm, Faculty of Health Sciences, University of Linkoping, Sweden.

References

Atkin, K. and Lunt, N. (1993) *Nurses Count: A National Census of Practice Nurses*. (Social Policy Research Unit: University of York).

Council for the Education and Training of Health Visitors (1977) *An Investigation into the Principles of Health Visiting*. (CETHV: London).

Department of Health (1990) *Caring for People: Community Care in the Next Decade and Beyond*. (HMSO: London).

Department of Health (1996a) *Choice and Opportunity: Primary Care – The Future*, Cmnd 3390. (HMSO: London).

Department of Health (1996b) *The Patient's Charter*. (HMSO: London).

Dimond, B. (1990) *Legal Aspects in Nursing*. (Prentice-Hall: Cambridge).

Dines, A. and Cribb, A. (1993) *Health Promotion Concepts and Practice*. (Blackwell Scientific: Oxford).

Downie, R.S. and Calman, K.C. (1987) *Healthy Respect: Ethics in Health Care*. (Faber and Faber: London).

Efstathiou, N. (1997) Personal communication. (Athens, Greece).

Kastana, S., Theodoropolou, P. and Theodoropolou, I. (1997) Personal communication. (Patras, Greece).

Harmen, H. (1996) For richer for poorer: the future of the NHS (Conference Address by the Shadow Secretary of State for Health) Association of Community Health Councils for England and Wales Conference: Harrogate.

Hunt, G. and Wainwright, P. (1994) *Expanding the Role of the Nurse*. (Blackwell Scientific: Oxford).

Knope, H. and Diekelmann, N. (1981) *Approaches to Teaching Primary Health Care*. (C.V. Mosby: St Louis).

Ministry of Social Affairs and Health (1996) *Health Care in Finland*. (Libris Oy: Helsinki).

Ministry of Social Affairs and Health (1997) *The Patient Injuries Act*. (Libris Oy: Helsinki).

National Statistical Office of Greece (1993) *Social Welfare and Health Statistics*. (Hellenic Republic NSSG: Athens).

Royal College of General Practitioners (1991) *Interprofessional Collaboration in Primary Health Care Organisations*. (RCGP: London).

Royal College of Nursing Institute of Advanced Nursing Education (1989) *Nurse Practitioner in Primary Health Care: Role Definition*. (RCNIANE: London).

Seedhouse, D. and Lovett, L. (1992) *Practical Medical Ethics*. (John Wiley & Sons: Chichester).

Svenska Institutet (1994) *General Facts on Sweden*. (FS 99z Nc: Stockholm).

Svenska Institutet (1995) *The Health Care System in Sweden*. (FS 99z Nc: Stockholm).

Thompson, I., Melia, K. and Boyd, K. (1988) *Nursing Ethics*, 2nd edn. (Churchill Livingstone: London).

Tope, R. (1996) *Integrated Interdisciplinary Learning between the Health and Social Care Professions*. (Avebury: Aldershot).

United Kingdom Central Council for Nurses, Midwives and Health Visitors (1992) *Code of Professional Conduct*, 3rd edn. (UKCC: London).

United Kingdom Central Council for Nurses, Midwives and Health Visitors (1996) *Guidelines for Professional Practice*. (UKCC: London).

World Health Organization (1995) *Annual World Health Statistics*. (WHO: Geneva).

Suggestions for further reading

Dines, A. and Cribb, A. (1993) *Health Promotion Concepts and Practice*. (Blackwell Scientific: Oxford).

Downie, R.S. and Calman, K.C. (1987) *Healthy Respect: Ethics in Health Care*. (Faber & Faber: London).

Gastrell, P. and Edwards, J. (eds) (1996) *Community Health Nursing: Frameworks for Practice*. (Baillière Tindall: London).

Mason, C. (ed.) (1997) *Achieving Quality in Community Health Care Nursing*. (Macmillan: Basingstoke).

Øvretveit, J., Mathias, P. and Thompson, T. (eds) (1997) *Interprofessional Working for Health and Social Care*. (Macmillan: Basingstoke).

Smith, H.L. and Churchill, L.R. (1986) *Professional Ethics and Primary Care Medicine*. (Duke University Press: Durham).

Wilmot, S. (1997) *The Ethics of Community Care*. (Cassell: London).

6

Ethical Issues in Maternity Care

Helen Crafter and Cathy Rowan

Introduction

This chapter will address some of the ethical issues in the delivery of maternity services which may have long-term repercussions on the health of women, children and families. In particular, attention is given to fetal screening tests and the issues surrounding the autonomy of both women and midwives during the process of birth. The role of the midwife in the United Kingdom (UK), Italy and Iceland will also be explored. Although the UK and Italy are in the European Union, maternity and midwifery practice in the two countries differ considerably. Iceland is not a member state of the European Union, but is a member of the European Free Trade Association (EFTA) which gives Icelanders the same freedom of movement as members of the European Union. Consequently, the education and training of midwives in Iceland comply with the EU Midwives Directives (see Appendix 1). The similarities and differences in maternity practices will be considered and salient points drawn together.

The ethical issues under scrutiny

The ethical issues surrounding birth have major repercussions for the world as a whole. As all of us are born and have, at least, a biological mother and father, so issues in pregnancy and birth are also pertinent to men. Half of the world's population are women and most women will give birth or be closely related to someone who does. The control a woman (and her partner) have over their lives, especially at such a monumental time as the birth of a child, must surely influence their feelings about themselves, their children and the world in which their children will grow, develop and perhaps raise their own families.

Fetal screening

Fetal screening tests are now routinely offered to women in Western Europe. The commonest are those for Down's syndrome and neural tube defects such as spina bifida and anencephaly. Many countries in the Mediterranean region or those with multicultural populations also offer haemoglobinopathy screening, particularly for thalassaemia or sickle cell disease, by offering blood tests to the parents.

Screening for fetal abnormalities is non-diagnostic but offers parents a risk ratio on which to consider whether they wish to proceed to more invasive diagnostic fetal tests such as amniocentesis. Probably the most widely used screening test throughout Europe is ultrasound scanning. It may be used to measure nuchal translucency (a measurement taken in the fetal neck region) and together with the fetal size and mother's age, can give a risk ratio for Down's syndrome at approximately 10–14 weeks of gestation. At present nuchal marker scanning will detect from 33 per cent (Nicolaides *et al.*, 1994) to 86 per cent (Bewley *et al.*, 1995) of fetuses with Down's syndrome. To a large extent, the reliability of the test depends upon the skill and experience of the operator and the quality of equipment available. Slightly later in the pregnancy ultrasound may be used to detect cardiac defects and duodenal atresia, both of which are associated with Down's syndrome. Approximately 40 per cent of babies with this abnormality have a cardiac malformation (Simpson, 1997a, p. 882) and 30 per cent of cases of duodenal atresia are associated with the condition (Simpson, 1997b, p. 914). Ultrasound scans therefore may be regarded as an ongoing screening process for Down's syndrome during the pregnancy.

Maternal serum screening for Down's syndrome calculates risk using a number of biochemical markers, most commonly alpha-fetoprotein (AFP), human gonadotrophin and unconjugated oestriols. The test is carried out between the 14th and 21st gestational weeks and, according to one UK study, will detect approximately 66 per cent of fetuses with Down's syndrome (North Thames West Region Institute for Medical Research, 1995). A risk of 1 in 250 or greater is regarded as 'screen positive' and the mother is likely to be offered a diagnostic amniocentesis. However, the actual odds of those with a positive screen result carrying an affected fetus is only 1 in 43 (Wald *et al.*, 1992). This suggests not only that there are a great many women who are left feeling anxious, but also a large number of amniocenteses are performed on the basis of an unreliable screening test. Furthermore, approximately 33 per cent of affected fetuses will be missed altogether following maternal serum screening, and even following excellent counselling, some couples may feel falsely confident that their unborn child is unaffected.

Alpha-fetoprotein screening for open neural tube defects has largely been abandoned in Western Europe in favour of diagnostic ultrasound scanning, which enables visualization of the abnormality. The AFP test performed at 16 to 18 weeks of gestation measures the protein which escapes from an open neural tube defect in the fetal spine or brain into the mother's bloodstream. A UK study (UK Collaborative Study on Alpha-fetoprotein in Relation to Neural Tube Defects, 1977) demonstrated that the test could detect 88 per cent of cases of anencephaly and 79 per cent of cases of open neural tube defect. However, it has been calculated that for every 15 women having an elevated alpha-fetoprotein level, only one will be carrying a fetus with a neural tube defect (Simpson, 1996, p. 225). Like the maternal serum screening test for Down's syndrome, the anxiety experienced by the large number of women who are given a false positive result can only be imagined.

'Haemoglobinopathy' refers to inherited abnormalities of haemoglobin in the red blood cells. In Europe the commonest of these are sickle cell disease and thalassaemia. Screening is again performed by parental blood testing if the mother carries the affected genes, so that the risk ratio for the fetus can be calculated. Sickle cell disease is seen mainly in people of African,

Caribbean, Mediterranean, Middle Eastern or Asian Indian origin, and thalassaemia in those of Mediterranean, Middle Eastern or South East Asian origin (Boyle, 1994). The practice of 'routine' haemoglobinopathy screening is growing throughout Europe, however, in response to inter-racial parenting and mass population movement.

Although fetal screening tests have been widely accepted as a positive move in antenatal care in many countries, their use confronts parents and health professionals with major ethical dilemmas. In their acceptance of screening tests, parents often see their purpose as confirming normality, whereas in the medical literature, doctors write of 'opportunities to investigate unborn babies for possible handicap' and 'identifying abnormalities early enough in pregnancy for termination to be feasible' (Whelton, 1990, p. 504). These incompatible objectives offer us some insight into the horror for the parents in being told that their risk ratio is higher than average and further tests, which will place their potentially normal child at risk (amniocentesis for instance carries a 1 per cent risk of miscarriage) should be considered.

The issue of informed choice in such circumstances is of great concern and it seems reasonable to ask, 'How can parents best be offered informed choice when they have little or no experience of children with the disability that their unborn child is being screened for?' This question is one of the hardest with which midwives and other health professionals at the sharp end of clinical practice have to deal. Even if a 'screen positive' result is followed up by diagnostic testing, the degree of affliction or disability often cannot be ascertained, especially in cases involving mental capacity.

There are also major concerns about the information and counselling available to parents prior to testing, especially bearing in mind that tests are usually offered at a time when the parents are still celebrating their luck at having conceived. Offering too little information may leave the parents unable to make an informed decision and in great shock if they screen positive. Too much information may frighten them into believing that the health professional considers them to be at additional risk. Either scenario may have negative repercussions on the parents' feelings of bonding with their unborn child or on their relationship with the health professionals involved in their care.

Women's right to autonomy

During labour and childbirth European women are also subjected to various routines, preferences and practices performed by health professionals in the name of 'safety', although these are often untested. These practices may be far removed from the admirable objectives of respecting women's choices and their right to self-determination and balancing these aims with the demands of evidence-based practice which is sensitive to women's needs and wishes. The publication of *Effective Care in Pregnancy and Childbirth* (Chalmers *et al.*, 1989) brought together the best of the systematic reviews into childbirth practices and makes salient reading for those of us who have subjected women to such unnecessary and unkind indignities as shaving pubic hair, having enemas while in labour and failing to provide continuity of care during pregnancy and childbirth.

Although evidence-based practice is a vital building block for safe and effective maternity care, it must take into account the psycho-social issues related to birth, as well as the rather dry and aloof results of randomized controlled trials which rarely take account of the individual needs of women and their families during the process of giving birth. Central to the debate surrounding evidence-based, humane childbirth are the issues of respect for women's autonomy and the degree of decision-making allowed her by the system in which she gives birth. An interesting measure of such autonomy is the extent to which women are given a choice about the place in which they give birth. In particular, the desire to deliver in the family home is one of the many important indications of who controls birth within a country's maternity service. In many European countries women have little choice in relation to the place of birth but are expected to comply with others' decisions about this fundamental aspect of the birth process.

The role of the midwife in Europe

Although the activities of a midwife, wherever she happens to reside, always involve caring for women and new-born infants at around the time of birth, the amount of responsibility held by midwives is largely determined by social tradition and the involvement of other professionals, particularly doctors, in maternity care.

Historically in Europe up until the seventeenth century, midwives, qualified only by their personal experience of birth, were the primary attendants. Doctors became increasingly involved after the industrial revolution and today an uneasy professional relationship exists between doctors and midwives as to the nature of their respective roles and where the boundaries of their respective professional activities meet.

When studying childbearing and early child-rearing practices in Europe it is readily apparent that the status of women in society and the role of the midwife are closely linked. Where childbirth is firmly under the control of doctors, so too is the practice of midwifery. The medical professional may also control the education of midwives, removing a powerful instrument through which midwifery can develop its own ethic and professionalism. In such countries pregnancy is treated in much the same way as illness. For example, a doctor's presence is considered necessary for antenatal care, the aim of 'care' is to diagnose abnormality and the woman's views are not highly valued in decisions about care management. Birth is conducted in hospital, the administration of drugs to the mother is commonplace, movement in labour is restricted and practices such as episiotomy and caesarean section are widespread. In countries where midwives have secured a more autonomous role, pregnancy is more likely to be viewed and treated as a normal life event. Antenatal care commonly takes place in the community under the jurisdiction of the midwife, the woman's psycho-social well-being is seen as important as her physical well-being and mechanisms are in place for women to give birth at home if they so wish.

However, even within the European Union where directives exist to protect women by formalizing the rules governing the practice of midwifery, their interpretation leads to a wide variation in the degree of professional autonomy which midwives possess. The European Midwives Liaison Committee (EMLC) (1996) produced a report of a study of the activities, responsibilities and independence of midwives in the 12 countries that were members of the European Union when the study began in the late 1980s. It was based on 3857 completed questionnaires received from chief midwives and midwives in clinical practice from nine European countries (Belgium, Denmark, France, Germany, Greece, the Netherlands, Ireland, Luxembourg and the United Kingdom.) No chief midwives in Italy, Portugal or Spain responded to the questionnaires and so the final report in its referral to these countries relied on data supplied by the few individual midwives who responded. This no doubt has a considerable effect on the reliability of the findings for those three countries.

The study gives a broad, if limited, picture of midwifery practice in Europe. Midwives appearing to have the greatest freedom and autonomy in decision-making were those in the Netherlands, France, Denmark and the UK, while those having the least were found in Belgium, Greece, Luxembourg and Portugal.

Considering that all midwifery practice in countries belonging to the European Union (EU) is controlled by the same European Economic Community (EEC) legislation (see Appendix), the existence of such wide variations in practice must have a complex multifactorial explanation, which is rooted in historical, cultural and political differences within each of the countries.

The value placed on women's autonomy

In the literature search which formed much of the background to preparing this chapter, the variations in midwifery practice, even in those countries governed by the EEC's Midwifery Directives, were staggering. Reading and hearing about women's expectations and experiences of maternity services proved equally enlightening, if somewhat disturbing. Some countries have well-established pressure groups, such as the National Childbirth Trust in the UK, while in other countries resignation, along with an almost complete trust of the medical model of childbirth, was apparent.

It is difficult to completely disentangle why and how countries, and even areas within them, acquire the maternity structures that exist. Is it because women truly do not care about how they give birth, so long as they and the baby are healthy? Is it because midwives by tradition are professionally weak, or is it because the medical profession is so much stronger? How is it that the psycho-social issues surrounding this most powerful emotional event are so often lost in the race to produce perfect children, at the perfect time, in a room full of strangers, who are more preoccupied with the latest technology than the woman's emotional well-being?

It is in the interests of humanity that children are born to women who are confident in their ability to carry, give birth to and nurture their infants. This is best achieved by listening to women and respecting their preferences in relation to pregnancy and the birth process, and also by not treating them like children by removing their responsibility and decision-making capacity at this sensitive time. All European countries are still recovering, to some degree, from the subordination of midwives to doctors which has been part of a general pattern of the medicalization of childbirth in which women are the recipients of maternity care, rather than active participants within it. To expect a labouring woman to submit to the so-called superior knowledge, expertise and whims of a professional group, most of whom have not experienced birth and motherhood themselves and then emerge as an assured and competent mother, is neither rational nor logical.

However, the autonomy of women during their childbearing and child-rearing periods is not a simple concept. Some women appear to be 'willing patients', happy to undertake whatever procedures their carers recommend for them. Some believe that safety is gained through technology and medical input and they expect these beliefs to be respected. Autonomy for women must begin well before they first become pregnant as truly informed choice is only available to women who are receptive to a broad range of information which acknowledges and deals with psycho-social, emotional and spiritual needs as well as physical ones. Women are, all after, products of their own cultural background and they continue to be influenced by these values throughout their whole lives.

The value placed on midwives' autonomy

But why should midwives be autonomous? Is it not safer for doctors to oversee the care of pregnant and labouring women and the training of midwives for that matter? Is it not safer to give birth in hospitals with access to emergency equipment in case things suddenly and unexpectedly go wrong?

There is increasing evidence from Europe and elsewhere that autonomous midwives who control their professional practice offer as safe an option for women and babies (Campbell and Macfarlane, 1994) or a safer one (Tew, 1995), as that offered when maternity services are overseen by doctors. Autonomous midwives also provide a service that leaves women more satisfied with the birth experience (Poulengeris and Flint, 1987; McCourt and Page, 1996). No-one would wish to deprive women of obstetric, anaesthetic and paediatric expertise where it is beneficial but, in the words of the Expert Maternity Group established in England by the Department of Health (1993):

A woman with an uncomplicated pregnancy should, if she wishes, be able to book with a midwife as the lead professional for the entire episode of care including delivery at a general hospital (p. 18)... The part which the midwife plays in maternity care should make full use of all her skills and knowledge, and reflect the full role for which she has been trained (p. 39)... The knowledge and skills of the obstetrician should be used primarily to provide advice, support and expertise for those women who have complicated pregnancies (p. 41).

The group also reinforced the finding of a Select Health Committee which reported in 1992:

On the basis of what we have heard, this committee must draw the conclusion that the policy of encouraging all women to give birth in hospitals cannot be justified on grounds of safety (p. 1).

At home births in Europe the midwife is necessarily the lead professional as the birth tends to be uncomplicated and a doctor, if present, is at risk of being called away to a patient with a medical ailment. The midwife working within the EU is duty bound to stay with the woman for the birth and the period immediately afterwards. It is difficult to imagine how a health worker who has not been entrusted with autonomy could effectively conduct a birth at home ensuring the safety, as well as the emotional well-being, of the family. The practice of Dutch midwives who are some of the most autonomous in Europe may be used here to demonstrate the value of midwives being the lead health care professional at the time of a birth. In Holland, approximately one-third of all births occur in the home yet the perinatal mortality rate is among the lowest in the world (Campbell and Macfarlane, 1994, p. 38). Indeed, a large Dutch study into 'place of birth' has demonstrated that for women having a first baby with a low-risk pregnancy, home birth is as safe an option as hospital birth. The same study also found that for multiparous women with a low-risk pregnancy, home birth was significantly safer than giving birth in hospital (Wiegers *et al.*, 1996). This finding, however, should be set alongside the activities of Dutch midwives who attend an extraordinarily high number of home births compared to midwives in the rest of Western Europe and who are, by experience therefore, extremely competent in dealing with births which occur in women's homes.

Ethical issues in maternity practices in the UK, Italy and Iceland

The EMLC (1996) reported through their survey of midwifery practice that UK midwives have a relatively higher level of autonomy than some of their European counterparts and Italian midwives less so. Icelandic midwives, while not in the EU, are governed by their midwifery rules, and practice is similar to that seen in the UK. Maternity services in Iceland, however, have not received the same governmental backing as those in the UK and concerns exist that the medicalization of childbirth in some areas is increasing rather than abating.

The United Kingdom

Health authorities vary throughout the United Kingdom with regard to the screening tests which may be offered to women. In some areas AFP screening is still routinely offered, while in others this has been replaced by diagnostic ultrasound scanning for open neural tube defects and anencephaly at 16–22 weeks of gestation. Unless a woman chooses private health care through an obstetrician or independent midwife all her maternity care, including screening tests, are paid for through the National Health Service (NHS). However, before its widespread introduction, some health authorities required women wishing to have the maternal serum screening test to pay for it. Part of the midwife's role is to inform women about the advantages and disadvantages of screening tests in an unbiased and non-judgemental way, as well as to support them by listening and providing further information once they have made a decision about availing themselves of the tests. Professional counsellors who may or may not be midwives are also available in some maternity units, particularly to support women who have screened positive and are considering the implications of the results.

The Midwives Information and Resource Service (MIDIRS) together with the NHS Centre for Reviews and Dissemination have recently produced a number of easily readable and understandable leaflets on 'Informed Choice' which provide information for women and health professionals based on the best available research evidence. Unfortunately these leaflets are only available in the English language and their dissemination is dependent upon health authorities purchasing them. To date, however, MIDIRS and the NHS Centre for Reviews and Dissemination have been delighted with the sales to NHS trusts (Rosser, 1996).

In the UK it is common, but by no means universal practice, for women to receive the majority of their antenatal care from a small team of midwives known to them by the time they go into labour. A guideline for future practice in the Department of Health *Changing Childbirth* report (1993) recommended that, by the year 1998, at least 75 per cent of women should know the midwife who delivers them. It seems unlikely, however, that this recommendation will be reached despite enormous changes to the regional organization of the maternity services (Mayes, 1997). One reason why it will not be achieved is the huge demand on NHS resources which cannot be met in the UK.

Almost all births take place in hospital but a further recommendation of the *Changing Childbirth* report (DoH, 1993) that women should receive clear, unbiased information and be able to choose where they would like their baby to be born may have paved the way for an increase in home births over the next decade as women and midwives strive to rekindle their confidence in choosing and attending home births.

Birth practices in the UK are far from being completely 'woman centred'. It is still common to see obstetricians patrolling delivery suites and managing childbirth as they would a medical ailment, even where women have a clearly written birth plan requesting minimal intervention and a midwife is competently attending the woman in a way that they both find acceptable. Induction of labour before 42 weeks of gestation in normal pregnancy and arbitrary limitation of the duration of the second stage of labour by performing an operative delivery are still not unusual procedures despite being listed as 'forms of care that should be abandoned in the light of the available evidence' (Chalmers *et al.*, 1989, p. 1477).

The education of student midwives is under the control of the profession but the recent move of departments of midwifery education into higher education, invariably into faculties of nursing, has meant that they are often headed by nurses. All midwifery training establishments must have an 'Approved Midwife Teacher' who formally leads the midwifery programmes, so that the departmental or faculty heads (nurses) tend to fulfil a purely administrative role. Midwives are educated to either diploma or degree level for three to four years. Alternatively, if they are already in possession of a registered general nurse qualification, they can gain a midwifery qualification in 18 months.

Italy

The Italian fertility rate is now among the lowest in the world (Council of Europe, 1996, p. 187). The fall began in the 1970s and in 1993 (the latest figure available) the total fertility rate was equal to 1.26 children per woman, giving a crude birth rate of 9.6 live births per 1000 average population (this may be compared to 17.5 for Iceland and 13.1 for the UK for 1993 [p. 41]). As well as having fewer children, couples are also bearing them at a relatively older age. This seems surprising in a country renowned for its large Catholic following, although it may be explained by Italy's recent modernization resulting in many more women working outside the home. This would not have been possible without access to contraception and the ability to plan a family to fit in with working practice. Although seen as desirable, children place enormous pressure on Italy's nuclear, urban families. The state provides little in the way of child support and child care facilities for working mothers and, as consumerism grows, couples choose to expand their luxury possessions rather than their families (Gumbel, 1997).

Despite the improving social status of women in modern Italy, pregnancy and birth are still heavily controlled by doctors. Fetal screening tests are commonplace and although a national health care system is in place, women pay extra for each test that they have. Ultrasound scanning tends to be offered (and unfailingly accepted) at 12, 20 and 34 weeks of gestation, and sometimes more frequently, to check for fetal viability, abnormalities and growth. Screening for neural tube defects and for Down's syndrome for women over 35 years of age is generally available.

On the Italian island of Sardinia, thalassaemia major is a common inherited disorder with a carrier frequency of 12.6 per cent, which means that one couple in every 60 is at risk of having an affected child. The incidence of the disease among new-born babies is 1 in 250 births (Cao, 1993). The condition has no cure and consequently a programme based on carrier screening, genetic counselling and prenatal diagnosis has commenced. Voluntary screening is offered to young unmarried adults, prospective parents and to couples where the woman is pregnant. Counselling is reported to be carried out according to internationally accepted guidelines. A large majority of women accept the prenatal diagnosis which is generally very accurate and many opt for termination rather than give birth to a child with a severely limited quality of life and lifespan.

Care and procedures for labour and birth differ greatly in Italian hospitals and birth is often supervised by doctors. Pain relief is rarely administered as the pain of labour is said to be a normal expectation for Italian women. Many hospitals offer muscle relaxants such as hyoscine in early labour and a few hospitals offer epidural analgesia, especially where a resident doctor has recently studied its administration abroad. Inhalational analgesia such as nitrous oxide 50 per cent and oxygen 50 per cent (commonly known under its trade name of 'Entonox' in the UK) is not used and pethidine and other narcotics are not readily available (Fracassi, 1997; Prevedello, 1997).

In 1984, Morrin reported on an observational visit to a maternity hospital near Rome. The labour rooms were communal and procedures such as vaginal examinations were performed with little privacy. Women laboured in a horizontal position and when full dilation of the cervix was diagnosed, the women were moved to their own room and instructed to bear down. A doctor was always present for the birth, episiotomy was used liberally and the infants were delivered by fundal pressure. These procedures are still practised in some parts of Italy (Frascassi, 1997; Prevedello, 1997). In some areas, particularly Tuscany, there is a more liberal approach towards birthing practices. Some hospitals have 'natural birth rooms' which are popular because women can walk around freely. In the maternity unit at Poggibonsi episiotomies are not performed unless strictly necessary and the midwife is responsible for the entire course of labour. Women's partners remain with them and the new-born baby is placed on the mother's abdomen, where the cord is cut only after it has stopped pulsating (Brunetti, 1993).

In theory Italian women have the right to home birth, but in much of the country the mechanisms are not in place for this to be a realistic possibility. Independent midwives exist and are cheaper to consult than their British counterparts. Their numbers appear to be growing as Italian midwives become increasingly concerned about their role in hospital births.

One of the reasons why birth is so medicalized in some parts of Italy may be explained by the role which doctors play in midwifery education. After two years in nurse education, student midwives study for another two years to qualify as a midwife. Throughout the country the midwifery programme is run by doctors who are involved in both developing and teaching the curriculum. The liberal use of episiotomy and delivery by fundal pressure are two major components of the programme and students may not see a physiologically normal birth throughout their whole period of training (Frascassi, 1997; Prevedello, 1997). The EMLC Report (1996) expressed concern about the deficient exposure of some student midwives to the full range of activities described in the EEC Directives and the implications for the ability of midwives trained in Italy to assume responsibility for the care of pregnant women, as required by EC statute. The problems of midwifery practice in Italy are compounded by the lack of an independent and competent midwifery authority for the country.

Iceland

In Iceland midwives are trained to an advanced clinical and theoretical level and on completion of their education are awarded both an educational certificate and a professional qualification. Since 1982 a nursing degree has been the level of entry. Eight midwives graduate a year from the 18-month midwifery programme at the University of Iceland which has been running in Reykjavik since January 1996. With the transfer of the programme to the university, midwives, for the first time, gained full control of their midwifery curriculum when a midwife was appointed as the Director of Midwifery Studies. Until this time the post had been held by a doctor (Olafsdottir, 1996). On qualification those who choose to practise midwifery join a workforce of 236 midwives who are involved in the 4500 births a year, two-thirds of which take place at the University Hospital of Iceland in Reykjavik.

Midwives attend almost all pregnant women although most also see a doctor on a few occasions, even when the pregnancy is uncomplicated. Most obstetricians and general practitioners still insist on seeing women at every antenatal visit and some women choose this medical approach to their care. The usual venue for antenatal care is in hospitals or health centres. There is no routine provision for antenatal care in women's homes. In many hospitals midwives perform and are responsible for routine ultrasonography which is offered to all women at 19 weeks' gestation. The midwives' role includes the provision of explanations and counselling. If a fetal abnormality is suspected on the scan the midwife cannot make a diagnosis or pass her concerns on to the woman. She must refer the woman to a specialist for a second opinion. AFP screening is offered to women who have a family history of spina bifida and those who request it, but it is not performed routinely. The test has, to a large extent, been superseded by diagnostic ultrasound imaging of the fetal spine and brain. The University Hospital of Iceland is likely to start offering maternal serum screening to women from the end of 1997 (Gottfredsdottir, 1997; Olafsdottir, 1997). In addition, women who reach their 35th birthday before the baby's due date are offered diagnostic amniocentesis at 14–16 weeks of gestation.

Iceland has a history of offering 'low risk' women birth centre care, which is characterized by a home-like environment and care by a small team of midwives. Such a birth centre existed in Reykjavik from 1960 to 1995, when, according to the media, it was closed for 'economic reasons'. The delivery rate at the centre declined rapidly following the opening of a large, high risk delivery unit in the University Hospital two miles away. This unit incorporated a birth unit staffed by six midwives with doctors only attending women when problems arise (Sigurdardottir *et al.*, 1996). The closure of the outlying birth centre where doctors had to travel the two miles to attend women and the setting up of the birth unit within the University Hospital have placed midwife-led care closer to medical jurisdiction and made the birth unit more vulnerable to hospital culture than was the community-based birth centre. There are also professional concerns from midwives about the effect that such proximity to medical involvement may have and the implications of this for the empowerment of women and midwives (Gottfredsdottir, 1997; Olafsdottir, 1997).

Continuity of carer schemes are not common and the prevailing policy is to centralize all maternity care. At the University Hospital where the majority of the country's births take place, midwives are department based rather than case-load based so that most women receive care from different midwives in pregnancy, labour and then postnatally.

Home birth is rare in Iceland. There are about 8–10 per year conducted by one midwife who offers these women care in labour and the post-partum period. Sometimes another midwife assists at the actual birth. The primary midwife stays with the woman booked for home birth if she requires transfer to hospital during labour. She has a contract with the state and like all Icelandic midwives is entitled to offer home birth and postnatal care and to claim expenses through the government health insurance system (Gottfredsdottir, 1997; Olafsdottir, 1997). The centralization of birth into hospitals has been the same in Iceland as in many European countries in recent times and the associated influence of a dominant medical profession in this shifting of childbirth from home into hospital has resulted in a transfer of decision-making about the birth process from both women and midwives alike.

The midwife is the leading professional for all normal births in Iceland and, as in most of Europe, doctors are readily available should medical assistance be necessary. In common with much of Europe and the United States, the normal delivery rate is slowly declining and caesarean and epidural analgesia rates are increasing in Iceland (Olafsdottir and Gottfredsdottir, 1996).

Conclusion

In Europe, women's experiences of childbearing are varied and they appear to depend, to a large extent, on the history of the health care professions, cultural preferences and political developments. The social status of women and the role of the midwife share many similarities and, where women are not encouraged to be active participants in decision-making, the role of the midwife also tends to be seen as subordinate to the medical profession.

Fetal screening tests are available in the UK, Italy and Iceland but who they are offered to and how women and couples are informed about their advantages and limitations varies considerably. In the UK screening tests are offered to almost all women and there is a move towards exploring how women can be provided with genuinely informed choices. In Italy screening and diagnostic testing are very popular especially in the large northern cities. The quality of information with which women are provided is, however, variable. The idea of 'counselling' in relation to such tests has different connotations from those that exist in the UK, with Italian counselling being more directive (Frascassi, 1997; Prevedello, 1997). In Iceland fetal screening tests, other than an ultrasound scan at 19 weeks of gestation and amniocentesis for women over 35 years of age, are not routinely offered, although maternal serum screening may be introduced in 1997/98.

Women's experiences of labour and birth are also diverse in Europe, despite the existence of EEC Midwives Directives designed to bring the activities of midwives into line across the European Union. Medical domination is apparent in all three countries in various ways. In Italy doctors preside over normal births in some maternity units and dictate that babies should be delivered by fundal pressure following the routine performance of an episiotomy, whereas this degree of intervention is not seen in the UK or Iceland. The mechanisms for home birth are in place in some areas of each country but the practice is not common and medical resistance continues. This is despite the support for women to have a home birth if they so wish, by governmental health departments, particularly in the UK and Iceland. As the evidence to refute the safety of home birth simply does not exist (Campbell and Macfarlane, 1994), the motivation of the medical profession to maintain control over normal birth must be questioned on the basis of whose interests are being served.

In our conversations with midwives from Italy and Iceland in the preparation of this chapter, we discussed the existence and role of women's groups in providing a supportive voice for the right to self-determination and a reduction in routine medical intervention in physiologically normal pregnancy and birth. The National Childbirth Trust in the UK provides a strong voice in commenting on these issues and it provided a sustained input during the compilation of the Department of Health (1993) *Changing Childbirth* report. However, our European colleagues explained that such pressure groups barely exist in Italy and Iceland. A group of women had attempted to keep the birth centre in Reykjavik open in the early 1990s, calling themselves the 'Children of Nature', but when the centre was closed despite their protest, the group disbanded. It is not clear why countries should have such varying experiences of pressure groups, but it may be that Italian and Icelandic women are more trusting of the medical profession, or less concerned about the psycho-social atmosphere in which they give birth.

Evidence-based practice too receives variable attention in different corners of Europe. The UK has a strong history of producing research and, as in the USA and Canada, there has been a strong push in recent decades to systematically review the available evidence and incorporate it into clinical practice. With the aim of developing practice that is known to increase good and reduce harm, it is likely that evidence-based care will spread throughout Europe resulting in many of the outdated and harmful practices being eventually eliminated. However, the vested interests of all health professionals must be put aside for this to happen and those of women and their families must finally be placed centre stage.

Acknowledgements

We wish to extend our thanks to Liliana Prevedello, Anna Frascassi, Helga Gottfredsdottir and Ardis Olafsdottir for their help in making this chapter possible.

References

Bewley, S., Roberts, L.J., Mackinson, A-M. *et al.* (1995) 'First trimester fetal nuchal translucency: problems with screening the general population 2', *British Journal of Obstetrics and Gynaecology*, **102**(5): 386–8.

Boyle, M. (1994) *Antenatal Investigations*. (Books for Midwives Press: Hale Cheshire).

Brunetti, A. (1993) 'Midwifery in Italy', MIDIRS *Midwifery Digest*, **3**(1): 16–17.

Campbell, R. and Macfarlane, A. (1994) *Where To Be Born? The Debate and the Evidence*, 2nd edn. (National Perinatal Epidemiology Unit: Oxford).

Cao, A. (1993) 'Preventing a genetic disease', *World Health*, **46**(6): 26–7.

Chalmers, I., Enkin, M. and Keirse, M.J.N.C. (1989) *Effective Care in Pregnancy and Childbirth*. (Oxford University Press: Oxford).

Council of Europe (1996) *Recent Demographic Developments in Europe*. (Council of Europe: Strasbourg).

Department of Health (1993) *Changing Childbirth Part 1: Report of the Expert Maternity Group*. (HMSO: London).

European Midwives Liaison Committee (1996) *Activities, Responsibilities and Independence of Midwives within the European Union*. (EMLC: Northampton).

Frascassi, A. (1997) Personal communication.

Gottfredsdottir, H. (1997) Personal communication.

Gumbel, A. (1997) 'Baby? I'd rather have a mobile', *Independent*, 2 March, p. 16.

Health Committee Second Report (1992) Session 1991–92: *Maternity Services*. (HMSO: London).

McCourt, C. and Page, L. (1996) *Report on the Evaluation of One-to-One Midwifery Practice*. (The Hammersmith Hospitals NHS Trust and Thames Valley University: London).

Mayes, G. (1997) Assistant Director for Midwifery Supervision and Practice, English National Board, personal communication.

Morrin, N. (1984) 'When in Rome', *Midwives Chronicle*, August, 260–1.

Nicolaides, K.H., Brizot, M.L. and Snijders, R.J.M. (1994) 'Fetal nuchal translucency: ultrasound screening for fetal trisomy in the first trimester of pregnancy'. *British Journal of Obstetrics and Gynaecology*, **101**(9): 782–6.

North Thames West Region (1995) *Maternal Serum Screening for Down's Syndrome and Open Neural Tube Defects: A Guide for Health Professionals*. (Harrow North West Thames Region Institute for Medical Research: London).

Olafsdottir, A. (1997) Personal communication.

Olafsdottir, A. and Gottfredsdottir, H. (1996) 'Are safety and economy justifiable reasons for the closure of birth centres?', unpublished MA essay. (Thames Valley University: London).

Olafsdottir, O.A. (1996) 'Midwifery studies in Iceland', International Confederation of Midwives 24th Triennial Congress Conference Proceedings, Oslo, May 26–31, p. 171.

Poulengeris, P. and Flint, C. (1987) The 'Know Your Midwife' Report, unpublished.

Prevedello, L. (1997) Personal communication.

Rosser, J. (1996) 'Informed choice – we have lift off!', *MIDIRS Midwifery Digest*, **6**(2): 142.

Sigurdardottir, C.N.M., Oladottir, S.M., Gudmundsdottir, P. *et al.* (1996) 'An alternative birth care unit in Reykjavik, Iceland', International Confederation of Midwives 24th Triennial Congress Conference Proceedings, Oslo, May 26–31, p. 114.

Simpson, C. (1997a) 'Cardiac and circulatory conditions in the newborn', in Sweet, B. and Tiran, D. (eds) *Mayes Midwifery*, 12th edn (Baillière Tindall: London), pp. 882–8.

Simpson, C. (1997b) 'Congenital malformations and conditions', in Sweet, B. and Tiran, D. (eds) *Mayes Midwifery*, 12th edn. (Baillière Tindall: London), pp. 912–20.

Simpson, J.L. (1996) 'Genetic counseling and pre-natal diagnosis', in Gabbe, S.G., Neibyl, J.R. and Simpson, J.L. (eds) *Obstetrics: Normal and Problem Pregnancies*, 3rd edn. (Churchill Livingstone: New York), pp. 215–48.

Tew, M. (1995) *Safer Childbirth? A Critical History of Maternity Care*, 2nd edn. (Chapman & Hall: London).

UK Collaborative Study on Alpha-fetoprotein in Relation to Neural Tube Defects (1977) 'Maternal serum-alpha-fetoprotein measurement in antenatal screening for anencephaly and spina bifida in early pregnancy', *Lancet*, **1**(25): 1323–32.

Wald, N., Kennard, A. and Densem, J. (1992) 'Antenatal maternal serum screening for Down's Syndrome: results of a demonstration project', *British Medical Journal*, **305**(3850): 391–4.

Whelton, J. (1990) 'Sharing the dilemmas – midwives' role in prenatal diagnosis and fetal medicine', *Professional Nurse*, July, 514–15.

Wiegers, T.A., Keirse, M.J.N.C., Berghs, G.A.H. *et al.* (1996) 'An approach to measuring the quality of midwifery care', *Journal of Clinical Epidemiology*, **49**: 319–25.

Suggestions for further reading

Abramsky, L. and Chapple, J. (eds) (1994) *Prenatal Diagnosis: The Human Side*. (Chapman & Hall: London).

Marland, H. (ed.) (1993) *The Art of Midwifery: Early Modern Midwives in Europe*. (Routledge: London).

World Health Organization (1996) *Care in Normal Birth: A Practical Guide, Report of A Technical Working Group*. (World Health Organization: Geneva).

7

Children, Rights and Nursing Concerns

Gosia Brykczynska

Introduction

Moral rights

Although philosophers have been commenting on matters of morality for several thousand years, it is only within the last few hundred years that a clear philosophical argument has been developed around the concept of moral rights. Writings on the nature of moral rights, what they are, who can lay claim to them, whom they benefit and what difference their existence makes to social morality – have been the preoccupation of Western philosophy since the time of John Locke (1632–1704). As Almond (1991) notes, although 'of comparatively recent vintage linguistically, rights belong to a tradition of ethical reasoning which goes back to antiquity. In relation to this tradition the overtones of the notion are legal rather than ethical.' Needless to say, this interest in rights, be they human, civil, political or social, is neither the sole prerogative of moral philosophers nor their sole interest. The literature on universal human rights has a long and fascinating history, the roots of which can be traced back to the doctrine of natural law, although it is only relatively recently that the rhetoric concerning rights and the popular understanding of them has entered the public domain. Today, therefore, it is not unusual to hear quite unsophisticated individuals demanding 'their rights' to parenthood, better housing, sovereignty and such like (Lumpp, 1982; Hart, 1984 [1967]). The fundamental questions remain, however: 'what are rights?', 'what do we mean by fundamental rights?', 'how do they impinge on health care?' and 'can a unique category of people, namely children, lay a particular claim to special rights?' This chapter will attempt to address these issues, within the context of paediatric nursing in Europe.

Rights have been varyingly described as claims that demand respect. Some rights demand more respect than others, such as the right to life, but even this seemingly obvious and uncontentious right is surrounded with qualifying clauses and commentaries. All humans can lay a claim to the right to live, providing, for instance, that they are already living, or that they have not forfeited that right by committing a capital offence, or that they are not deemed to be living in a state which is itself incompatible with life and so on. If the 'right to life' is potentially as problematic as this, it is not difficult to imagine that many other rights of presumably lesser significance will be even more contentious. Any reasonable definition of a right, or rights, needs to acknowledge the relative nature of any set of rights. The definition of a right as a claim that demands respect, while fairly basic and therefore quite useful, has of course the in-built limitation that it does not accord that right any obvious hierarchical standing or make clear the extent or limit of the respect due. Historically, rights were seen and considered as personal or political claims concerning one's freedom (that is, autonomy) which demands the respect of an autocratic ruler. Such an approach was taken in the writings of John Locke (Waldron, 1984).

The first philosophers writing about human rights were, for the most part, concerned with what today would be referred to as political and social rights. They were not particularly concerned with all people, that is, all of humanity, but rather the specific rights of a certain set of people, nor were they particularly concerned that their theories about claims that deserve respect were limited and narrow. Nonetheless, there is a direct line of philosophical argument concerning rights which stems initially from the political philosophies of David Hume and John Locke, through the French and American writers, such as Jean

Jacques Rousseau and Benjamin Franklin, all of whom influenced the course of American and French philosophical history, down to the present day. As a result of this historical legacy, both France and the United States of America, even today, see themselves as custodians and inheritors of the notion of human rights, even though, in recent times, neither country has produced significant new contributions to the philosophical debate on rights. In keeping with the rest of contemporary Western society, these countries are, however, concerned with the implementation of various rights. In the case of the United States of America, while it has a history of producing Charters and Bills of Rights (both specific and general), it has paradoxically a less illustrious history of implementing these rights. The widespread impact of the unprecedented violations of human rights which occurred during the Second World War led to the signing of the United Nations' Declaration of Human Rights in 1948.

The rights in which we are interested as health care workers are those that demand respect in relation to promoting, restoring and maintaining health. Additionally, in paediatric nursing and child health care, these claims will be child centred. Beauchamp and Childress in their highly influential textbook on biomedical ethics (1989) make the additional qualification with regard to rights, that they are justifiable claims. They point out that 'A right is thus analogous to property over which one has control, so that rights contrast with privileges, personal ideals, optional acts of charity, and the like (p. 56).

Health care rights

In the context of health care, one of the most fundamental rights to which a person can lay a justifiable claim, is the right to personal involvement in treatment – otherwise known as a right to autonomous decision-making about one's care, or at least a fairly shared decision-making process and some involvement (Brazier and Lobjoit, 1991; Kultgen, 1995). This right tends to take precedence over other related health care rights because most other rights, such as the right to a particular type of treatment or medical intervention, can be seen as a form of personal ideal such as the right to bear children, or the right to an organ transplant. The inherent problem with the rights debate is that one person's right is another person's ideal, fancy or act of charity. Rights, therefore, tend to be seen as having prima facie considerations, that is, they are only morally binding if no other, more pressing, claim is evident. Similarly, health care rights are only binding insofar as a more morally binding right does not take precedence (Lumpp, 1982; Reckling, 1994). Regardless of the inherent or relative value of a rights claim, it should ideally be something over which an individual can have control or do something about, such as the example of property given by Beauchamp and Childress (1989). This distinction is important and is a source of much misunderstanding as it is nonsensical to demand respect in relation to a claim that, although justifiable in itself, cannot be ordinarily realizable, as for instance, the right to a heart transplant. One can make a justifiable claim concerning equal access to transplant services, but not that a particular organ be provided, since there is no moral or legal way of assuring a guaranteed availability of such an organ. Neither health care workers nor society generally has control over this commodity and, therefore, such a right has no realizable obligation (Emson, 1992). In effect, we have no control over the availability of organs for transplantation. It is interesting to note here that in a case concerning the demand of a leukaemic patient that his cousin be obliged to donate his bone marrow to save his life, the judge commented that although the cousin could not be forced to give his bone marrow, the fact that he refused to help his cousin said much about his lack of moral integrity. In that particular case, the judge, confirming the thinking of much of society, agreed that whereas there is no right to an organ transplantation and life-saving measures, society still has a moral obligation to facilitate life-saving measures whenever it can do so (Beauchamp and Childress, 1994, p. 192).

Health care rights are often quite complex and multifactorial because, although health and health maintenance can often be seen as a shared responsibility between an individual and society, this is not always that obvious. For example, in the case of individuals with congenital disorders, the right to health *per se* and the right to have health restored is even more problematic. One cannot respect a claim to health *per se*, since we have limited control over matters of health and there are too many variables and unknowns at stake. We can, however, and indeed do, have a moral obligation to strive for conditions that promote health, allow individuals to stay healthy and so on (Lumpp, 1982; Hart, 1984 [1967]; Emson, 1992).

If society acknowledges, often through legislation, that certain universal rights, namely subsistence rights, such as a guaranteed access to health care facilities, the right to sufficient and appropriate food, or the right to shelter, do exist, then it is also acknowledging that, as a society, it has an obligation to intervene in respecting those rights. In other words, it has an obligation to act in a particular way. Traditionally, the correlativity of rights and obligations was such that everyone benefited from the recognition of certain basic rights and, therefore, the burden of the obligation to respect these rights served everyone's interest. Such arguments were possible, however, only in societies which acknowledged very few rights, for example, the right to vote, to own property and the right to mobility within a country. All citizens can be seen to benefit from such rights. The more a society increases its rights, however, the more likely it is that some of the rights will place burdens or obligations on citizens which are far removed from any obvious secondary benefits. Not only does this put a potential strain on the society as a whole, but members are more likely to object that the additional rights are not justifiable and, since all rights have only a prima facie force behind them, these additional rights will be increasingly disregarded or deemed of low significance. In effect, they will be rights on paper only because other, more universally pressing and obvious rights will be taking precedence (Ackerman, 1991). This is not merely an academic debate, conducted for the satisfaction of moral philosophers and social policy-makers, rather these are very serious limitations of the rights approach to social inequities and these same limitations seriously affect the outcome of a rights-based approach to health care ethics (Upton, 1993).

The questions must be posed, 'why engage in a rights-based approach to health care?' and 'why are the affairs of children so closely tied up with children's rights?' Traditional approaches to moral philosophy and ethical conduct tend to emphasize the moral obligation of the agent to behave in a particular way. Whether following a deontological or consequentialist form of argument, the moral theory ultimately supports a need for increased virtue and an awareness of moral responsibility. Whereas this primary virtue-based approach is necessary for personal moral development, it does not always address the problems and needs manifest through moral injustices, moral distress and ethical dilemmas (Upton, 1993). Some problems seem to be on a large scale or dimension and a purely personal approach, represented by virtue ethics and a particular philo-sophical orientation, does not seem to resolve them. Some social, political and moral injustices cannot be corrected by a purely personal approach. Thus, moral philosophers commenting on social injustices arrived at the notion that certain ways of human being or human conduct are necessary for universal human happiness and that these ways of being should, therefore, be guaranteed for everyone (Hart, 1984 [1967]; Waldron, 1984). So fundamental were these self-evident truths that to violate or transgress these rights incurred much moral condemnation and, eventually, they were reinforced by legal sanctions.

Rights-based approaches to ethical issues can be seen, there-fore, as generalizable forms of accepted moral norms, in circumstances where personal ethical approaches may not suffice and, even if they did, they would relegate moral conduct to the realm of optional choice (Warnock, 1992). Some moral ways of being are simply deemed too important to be left to chance. Additionally, as noted, some social and moral injustices can only be corrected by a concerted societal approach (Rawls, 1971; Leach, 1994). Thus, no one indi-vidual can assure access to health care, but a country's legis-lation reflecting the right of access to health care can begin to address this problem. Perhaps the simplest way to describe the two approaches is that, whereas a virtue-based ethical orientation tends to reflect personal choice, a rights-based approach reflects societal choice or preference. Personally, I may think it important to respect all individuals as best as I know how, but it is a societal norm and expectation that all citizens will be accorded the right to equal opportunities and employment policies. Such examples are not difficult to consider and all rights can be translated into classical ethical propositions. These approaches complement each other, rather than reflect opposing perspectives.

Children's rights

So far we have discussed rights generally without considering the issue of children's rights. This is quite appropriate as the literature and arguments for children's rights stem from and owe their origin to the general movement concerning human rights. Indeed, some individuals believe that children should not be accorded separate rights as these already exist as general rights accorded to all individuals, including children. There is some merit to this argument, but because of the vulnerable status of children, most countries have felt it necessary to either accord children separate rights or at least to articulate their rights in a special place so that they are not subsumed among general rights (Archard, 1993; Alston, 1994).

The history of children's rights is closely connected with the history of childhood, that is, as the evolving concept of childhood took shape, so too did the concept of children's rights (Stainton and Stainton, 1992; Archard, 1993; Brykczynska, 1993; Matthews, 1994). First of all, however, one needs to 'see' children, before one can accord them any rights. Not only is it important to 'see' children, but one needs to appreciate children in a state of childhood before one can start to consider any rights, obligations or moral norms in respect of this rather heterogeneous group of individuals, who may be united solely by the fact that their respective governments consider them to be politically under age, that is, they are denied the right to vote. Until a few years ago, there was no global unifying definition of childhood; now with the United Nations Children's Convention, there is at least a minimal definition of a child, as an individual below the age of legal and political majority, which can vary from 17 to 21 years.

Philosophers have long considered children as incomplete adults, that is, not only as smaller versions of adults, a concept not unique to philosophy but one shared by society as a whole, but also as adults in the making. This of course is partially true, as in due course children do become adults. The interesting factor about childhood, however, is not that it is a transitional stage between birth and adulthood, but that it is a fascinating time of varying length, worthy of consideration in its own right and hardly a primarily transitional phase (Matthews, 1994). Childhood needs to be experienced and lived through by children as a time appropriate for them. As such, it has intrinsic and not just relational or secondary value.

The importance of childhood cannot be overestimated, the more thoroughly childish and child-centred the childhood, the better prepared the child will be for adulthood. Commentators on childhood such as David Archard (1993), Gareth Matthews (1994) and Penelope Leach (1994) all concur that many adults, by forgetting what it was like to be a child, assume that it was an insignificant time in their life. All the child-centred evidence appears to suggest that as childhood is now and not transient for children, it is of supreme significance for them. Notwithstanding the psychological origins of childhood amnesia, the problem does remain that if being a child is such a difficult and stressful time, how come children seem to grow out of this, and forget the pain? Contemporary child psychologists, developmentalists and health care workers all point out that children do not really 'forget' the pain or joys of childhood, but rather, the trials, tribulations and activities of childhood shape and inform the moral and social integrity of the emerging adult.

Child activists claim that by not taking the child seriously, by for example, dismissing their concerns because they are fleeting and often oddly phrased to the adult's way of understanding, we are not only doing children a disfavour, if not grave injustice, but we are also denying part of our own personal history. We were all children once, we reacted and spoke like children and we contributed to the adult world like children. Childhood amnesia may have contributed to adults forgetting about their own childhood memories, but children living today need to be accorded respect like all members of society – a respect that overrides the adult's veil of childhood memory. Fortunately, some adults manage to remember what it was like to be a child and they have a passionate interest in helping children to live fruitful and joyful childhoods. These adults are some of the most vociferous campaigners for children's rights.

One of the earliest campaigners for the recognition of children's rights was Dr Janusz Korczak. Korczak (1878–1942) was probably one of the most legendary figures to emerge from the Holocaust, barring the adolescent diary-writer, Anne Frank (Lifton, 1988). Janusz Korczak, the *nom de plume* of Doctor Henry Goldszmit, was a child psychologist, paediatrician, educator, writer (for adults and children) and above all, a believer in children. His ideas concerning children's abilities, their insights and the way we should respect and relate to them, are only now being rediscovered and promoted (Newell, 1989; Alderson, 1993; Leach, 1994). To give final witness to his trust and care for children, he chose to stay with them rather than leave them to their fate in the Warsaw ghetto and, from there, he and the children were taken to be gassed by the Nazis in 1942.

More recently, Matthews in the United States of America and Priscilla Alderson in the United Kingdom, represent concerned individuals who are striving to improve the way adults think about and treat children (Alderson, 1993; Matthews, 1994). According to Matthews, an American philosopher, children have the natural capacity to ask the obvious question and to process the most unusual or uncommon answer, an ability which adults tend to lose. A child will seriously want to know why the world is round or where words come from and steadfastly stay with the answer – as long as they can process it. Matthews' book *The Philosophy of Childhood*, like his previous study, is peppered with examples of children asking philosophical questions and energetically engaging in philosophical debate, as his wonderful discussion on the nature of the universe illustrates (Matthews, 1994, pp. 10–12). Children have the delightful capacity to appreciate explanations, process these and accommodate the answers according to their cognitive abilities. As Matthews states about himself, 'I can't remember asking myself, as a child what time is. But I did puzzle over the beginning of the world' (p. 13). This innate capacity of children to ask fundamental questions about the world in which they live is part of their richness and intellectual wealth – a treasure lost by many adults. As Matthews points out, according rights to children is not a paternalistic or parentalistic act, it is simply acknowledging the debt adults owe children. Children are not only 'takers'. Even at an early age, children are capable of giving and delighting adults and sharing in the common heritage that is meaningful human interaction (Darbyshire, 1989; Montgomery, 1993; Worswick, 1993; Edwards, 1996).

Priscilla Alderson has long been a campaigner for increased children's rights, particularly in relation to health care. As she points out '... children in hospital have certain autonomy rights, but schools deny basic rights to their pupils and are imposing unprecedented amounts of compulsory tests and curriculum subjects on them. Parents, not children, are perceived as the consumers of education' (Alderson, 1993, p. 31). This observation, that the rights we accord to children are haphazard and in any event are there to serve adults rather than children, is a point which is highlighted by many advocates of genuine rights for children. As a teacher and mother, Alderson began her interest in children's rights and the legal aspects of their status when she was studying parental consent for surgery (Alderson, 1990). This first-hand familiarity with children, like Matthews and Korczak before him, has led these and many other children's rights' advocates to the conclusion that children need to be accorded rights because their interests are not being served by general rights, proclamations and universal laws. Also, children are demonstrating, and probably always have, more rationality and discernment than is allowed by the casual dismissal of children as immature, cognitively unstable or incapable of decision-making and reflection (Montgomery, 1993; Alston, 1994; Dimond, 1996; Hendrick, 1997).

Children's rights began to be seriously debated at the conclusion of the Second World War by the Human Rights Committee – who, in 1959, drew up the United Nation's Declaration of Children's Rights. This declaration was in force until the International Year of the Child, hosted by UNICEF in 1979. In Poland, in order to highlight his contribution to children's rights, 1978 was designated as the centenary year commemorating the work and life of Janusz Korczak. As a (then) communist country, Poland was also keen to make a public statement which would be listened to by Western powers. Thus, the Polish delegate to the United Nations (UNICEF) chose that year to call for a review of the Declaration of Children's Rights, which was neither widely known, nor had any force of law worth speaking of. From 1979 to 1989, the new Convention of Children's Rights was drafted repeatedly until finally, on 20 November 1989, the United Nations Convention on the Rights of the Child was circulated to countries for ratification. In all, 172 countries have ratified it, the highest number of ratifications of any international human rights treaty. The United States of America was one of the last countries to sign the ratification document, the United Kingdom doing so in December 1991. The conception, wording, acceptance ratification, final declaration and launch of the Convention, at the Children's Summit in New York City in September 1990, was dogged by (adult) controversy, acrimony and infighting. Notwithstanding all of the problems contingent on the production of the Convention, it is now part of the universal heritage of all children.

The United Nations Convention on Children's Rights

The United Nations Convention on Children's Rights is a collection of 54 articles which collectively outline those rights which the universal adult world deems necessary for the maintenance of children's self-esteem and autonomy. The articles are presented in groups related to various areas of a child's life and some have more moral force behind them than others. Probably the single, greatest criticism of the Convention is that although it has the status of international law, national laws concerning children take precedence, at least in the first instance (Alston *et al.*, 1992; Rogers and Roche, 1994). In the United Kingdom, the Children's Convention informs public policy concerning children but it is the Children Act 1989 that actually guides social action and social policy. Complaints of infringements of the Children's Convention can be addressed to the Court of Human Rights in Strasbourg, as can complaints about violations of the Children Act 1989. Even before the launch of the Children's Convention, however, the Parliamentary Assembly of the Council of Europe passed a resolution in 1986, termed the *Resolution of the European Parliament on a Charter for Children in Hospital*, several points of which are still not adhered to today (Rosenbaum and Newell, 1992). The principles, such as the right of every child to life from the moment of conception, to shelter, to be recognized as needing a nurturing environment, to protection from abuse of drugs, smoking, alcohol and such like, are still not binding in the European community, nor are they part of the 1989 Children Act in the United Kingdom (Newell, 1991). In May 1988, members of 12 European countries formalized a statement concerning children in hospital and drew up a European Charter for Children in Hospital.

Finally, the National Association for the Welfare of Children in Hospital (NAWCH) in the United Kingdom, now renamed Action for Sick Children (ASC), launched its charter concerning the rights of children in hospital. All these charters and documents, however well intended, do not have the full force of the law behind them. Therefore, should it be proven that some other more pressing issues have precedence over a claim concerning a child's rights, there is no power to change or alter this understanding (Rosenbaum and Newell, 1992). Hope for children stems from the monitoring facilities put into place by UNICEF, in relation to implementing the spirit of the United Nations Convention on Children's Rights. The first report, prepared by the monitoring task force in February 1994, severely criticized the United Kingdom government of the day for not doing enough to implement the spirit of the Convention or to publicize its articles (UNCRC, 1995).

As Brigit Dimond (1996) points out, 'even though at present they have no statutory force, the articles should be the basis of the purchase and provision of child health services' (p. 6). The rest of this chapter will focus on the four main articles of the United Nations Convention of Children's Rights which relate to health care work, and using examples from European countries, it will explore how children's rights in this area are respected and put into practice. Even prima facie rights have to be enforceable sometimes if they are to be considered as rights and not just pleasant sentiments or desires.

Article 12

> The child has a right to express an opinion and to have that opinion
> taken into account, in any matter or procedure affecting the child.

This is one of the most frequently cited articles in the Children's Convention and is reflected in a similar point made in the United Kingdom's (1989) Children Act. It is difficult to appreciate just how fundamental this right is, given that adults assume that it is their prerogative to have an opinion and to voice their concerns. In fact, it could be seen as a definition of adulthood that an adult is a person who can voice his or her opinion and that this opinion will be respected. Adults do not need to refer to someone who is older or even wiser. Adults are deemed mature enough, unless proven otherwise, to state their opinions and make their own private and public choices. As Mary Warnock (1992) comments, 'one of the major factors which can inhibit our freedom and diminish our power to choose is not age or poverty, but simply the role bestowed on us by other people who wish us, puppet-like, to play the scene their way' (p. 231). According to many child developmentalists and advocates of children's rights, the reason why we do not hear what children have to say is that we accord them a voiceless role in a play where adults write the script. Since children traditionally have been considered voiceless on matters that counted, children were never consulted. Decisions were made in the best interest of the child, according to the prevailing paediatric theory at the time. Since children's opinions were not solicited, no-one knew for sure how children felt about decisions. They were, like the old adage, literally seen but not heard. This position has changed recently with the ratification of the Children's Convention. Now it is public social policy that children's views are solicited. Whether this will result in a major change in our attitude towards children it is too early to state definitely, but certainly, children are to be consulted, their opinions noted and, wherever possible, their statement of preferences appropriately acted upon.

Priscilla Alderson (1993) in her brilliant study on children's capacity to consent to surgery, notes that, 'young patients suffer double discrimination as patients and also as children. The qualities attributed to adult patients: ignorance, inexperience, too much emotion, too little rationality, helpless dependence, are also attributed to childhood' (p. 9). The voice that is now given over to children is not only the frightened cry of an infant, a cry usually of meaningful protest, as Ulla Fasting (1995) the Danish paediatric nurse notes. It is, as Alderson (1993) identifies, the more rational protest of the school-age child and the active participation and co-operation of the adolescent. That children should have a say in matters that concern them is now a universal requirement contingent on implementing the articles of the Children's Convention. In Europe, different countries approach this point in different ways.

France

In France, child lawyers recognize the need to work with children and gain their co-operation as a defensive move lest children start to demand their right to be consulted and heard, if not in France itself, then at the Court of Human Rights in Strasbourg. Jacqueline Rubellin-Devichi (1994), a French lawyer who specializes in child and family law, in an interesting essay on the understanding of the principle of best interests of a child, enshrined in Article 3 of the Convention of the Rights of the Child, comments that 'the [French] legislature was well aware of the need to pass implementing legislation quickly so as to avoid the humiliation of a moral sanction and even a possible legal sanction by the European Court of Human Rights on the basis of a violation of the child's human rights'. In France, the National Assembly is in the process of addressing itself to the passing of child-centred laws covering three main areas related to childhood, children and family law, namely – issues of parentage, inheritance and divorce. According to Rubellin-Devichi (1994), some progress has been made but the main obstacle to according children the rights acknowledged in the Convention, especially the right to be heard, is that 'the French, convinced that parents know best what is good for their children, tend to consider that parents are better placed than the children themselves to discern their aspirations, their interests, as well as to defend their rights' (Rubellin-Devichi, 1994).

This deep-seated parentalism is not unique to the French, but as Rubellin-Devichi's essay clearly illustrates, it is national and cultural norms that are challenged by the insistence that age-old customs be waived in preference to new ideologies, however commendable the new ideology. In France, up until recently, the problem in upholding Article 12 of the Convention was that children could not initiate a legal case, in fact, they could not appoint their own lawyer. As recently as 12 June 1992, the Court of Appeal of Colmar (Jurisdata No. 41760) threw out of court the case of a child who wished to challenge the decision of a lower court on the grounds that there is no child-centred 'specific implementing legislation'. However, as of 8 January 1993, the new French children's law will allow for a child to have a formal voice in legal affairs concerning its own welfare. As in the United Kingdom, paediatric nurses in France need to understand the spirit of their new national laws and the spirit of the Children's Convention with which the French laws are trying to comply. As is often noted, the United Nations Convention on Children's Rights takes precedence over local laws and local laws must try to comply with the Convention!

In health care practice in France, as in the United Kingdom, allowing or even encouraging a child to have a say about treatment modalities, agreeing and consenting to medical interventions, as well as assenting to various health care protocols, are all expected under the Children's Convention. However, as Alderson (1993) comments, it is not legislation that is holding children up, but the attitude of adults towards children. She states, 'the key to respect for children's rights is respect for their rationality' (p. 40) and respect for a child's rationality is more an ethical and cultural value than something primarily enshrined in law (Montgomery, 1993).

Article 19

The state has an obligation to protect children from all forms of maltreatment perpetrated by parents or others responsible for their care, and to undertake preventive and treatment programmes in this regard.

It is customary to regard maltreatment of children as something that other people do to youngsters. It is difficult for health care workers to imagine that they may be contributing to a child's distress. Apart from the obvious instances where health care workers physically harm children, such as female genital mutilation, male circumcision or the sad case of Beverley Allitt, a British-born enrolled nurse, who within a four-month period managed to kill four children in her care and harm several others (Department of Health, 1994), there are many examples of psychological harm and harm inflicted on the maturing psyche of the child, of which sexual abuse is one example. The maltreatment that is focused on less frequently and one that is quite topical in Europe, especially Central Europe, is the harm inflicted on children by the way that they are treated in hospital. According to Ulla Fasting from Denmark, however, the crime that health care workers perpetrate on children is much more pervasive and much more subtle, but it is possibly just as devastating for the child (Fasting, 1995). The 'new' iatrogenesis she refers to is the infringement of the child's physical and psychological integrity by modern medicine and biotechnical prowess. She is especially concerned about the consequences (as yet only poorly researched) of *in vitro* fertilization techniques on the developing embryo and the effects of technology on the premature infant. Ulla Fasting, a paediatric nurse from Vyborg, Denmark, has for many years campaigned for a more child-centred approach to intensive care units. For a number of years at Danish conferences, she has outspokenly defended the right of a child not to be constantly prodded, pricked, turned, naso-gastrically fed and so on. The very technology that was set in place to save small children is now the cause of much of their distress. In fact, if health care workers do not heed the warnings of activists like Ulla Fasting they will be guilty of knowingly inflicting harm, a point emphasized by English neonatal nurse colleagues (Whyte, 1989; Crawford and Morris, 1994). This essentially iatrogenic understanding of harm perpetrated on children is a concern occupying the hearts and minds not only of physicians and nurses in the United Kingdom, but also of those in the poorer, new democratic countries of Europe, where only now are health care workers reading the relevant literature on psychological damage to children in hospitals.

Poland

The state is obliged to protect children from harm. The mandate here includes health care workers increasing their sensitivities regarding potential abuse of children and the state putting relevant bodies and mechanisms in place to deal with the consequences of abuse. If child abuse is not recognized and there is no reporting agency or laws to deal with the maltreating adults, then Article 19 has little local significance (Newell, 1991; Alston, 1994). The recent widely publicized scandals of paedophile rings in Belgium, Holland and England serve to highlight the pervasiveness of sexual abuse of children. If paedophile rings are so widespread and involve so many men (and women), it is not surprising that some nurses will also be paedophiles – as will some physicians (Long, 1992). These examples occur in all countries and certainly it is the declared aim of all European countries to curb and eradicate such organized crime.

In Central Europe, in addition to any harm inflicted as a result of abuse, or the 'new' iatrogenesis spoken of above, is the deep psychological trauma experienced by children who have to go to hospital, usually for long periods of time, without the support of parents or relatives. Although some more progressive centres are inviting parents, especially mothers, to stay with a child in hospital, this is still a relatively rare phenomenon. The greatest obstacle to changing the status quo is not necessarily entrenched positions of paediatricians, who often travel abroad and read foreign medical journals and would not mind changing set ways, but the inflexible position of Ministries of Health which produce directives concerning these matters. All too often objections are also raised by paediatric nurses themselves who are poorly and inadequately trained and feel threatened by parents staying on the wards. Needless to say, this is not the position everywhere and centres of paediatric excellence exist all over Central Europe. However, until more nurses are educated in a holistic fashion with input from child psychologists, child developmentalists and play leaders, it will be very difficult to change the fate of children in hospital wards. In Poland and Romania, paediatric nurses not only have newly founded organizations wherein to voice their concerns, but in Poland they now have a special three-year, part-time, post registration programme in paediatric nursing running at two sites.

Recently, Polish paediatric nurses pushed for the translation of several child development and child psychology textbooks, including a book on ethical issues in paediatric nursing. Brykczynska's (1989) text on ethical issues in paediatric nursing is now compulsory reading on the new nursing programmes. Similarly, the Hungarian nursing centre for continuing education in Budapest has helped publish the translation of Benjamin and Curtis's (1992) textbook on nursing ethics. Such concerted activity in the spirit of Article 19 can only bode well, even if there is still a long way to go in recognizing that health care workers themselves may be contributing to the fears and distresses of children.

Article 23

Handicapped children have a right to special care, education and training designed to help them to achieve a greater possible self-reliance and to lead a full and active life in society.

The United Kingdom

In the United Kingdom, children are considered, at least theoretically, sufficiently equal that neither ethnic origin, genetic predispositions, chronic disease nor infirmity should make a difference with regard to the treatment they may require. In practice, however, children with handicapping conditions, whether they are all embracing, such as severe multiple handicaps, or confined to only one or two areas such as dyslexia, visual or hearing impairment or chronic diseases such as diabetes or cerebral palsy, find that access to comprehensive child-centred services is neither easy nor automatic and equitable. The United Kingdom has several laws in place guaranteeing access to health, education and appropriate social services for children. The problem is not the lack of good intention and understanding of the need for better services for children, but the lack of adequate resources.

Although children comprise approximately a quarter of the United Kingdom population, they do not have a quarter of the available health care budget. Child-centred services, which are highly specific and therefore expensive, are both more costly per child patient in proportion to similar treatment for an adult, but are often inadequate or overly compromising and scarce. This was one of the contributing factors operating behind the scenes that made Beverley Allitt's conduct possible (Department of Health, 1994). In effect this means inequitable distribution of paediatric services over the country as a whole. Even if a child can have relatively good in-patient care, there is no assurance that the child will have appropriate community care. The advent of internal markets, the separation of community and acute service trusts, along with a jostling for increased funding from local services, has resulted in social and community health services working with separate budgets, and therefore the child in the middle often loses out on comprehensive co-ordinated care. It is too early to state whether this situation will be resolved, certainly the idea that government monies will follow the child has not materialized and there is much evidence that the available services for handicapped children are piecemeal rather than part of a comprehensive service. Most disturbing of all is that the type of care and care package a child gets depends on where a child lives. Geography seems to determine the availability of services rather than basic health needs. Perhaps this was always the case, but now it is much more blatant and the differences far more obvious. Presumably, some children always had better access to hospitals, paediatric consultants or nursing homes, but now some children have no access to community paediatric nurses, paediatric nursing homes or certain aspects of paediatric social services as these services do not exist in certain areas because they are not seen as a sufficiently high priority to be guaranteed for all children who might need them. The result of such inequity is that some children have a disproportionately better start in life, despite their handicaps, than other children. There is also evidence that some ethnic groups are simply not engaging in the paediatric services, even when they are available (Slater, 1993).

Central Europe

On the continent of Europe, for the most part, finances follow the child and paediatric services are, at least theoretically, more co-ordinated. Countries of the old communist bloc had highly developed child-centred services and children with handicapping conditions had access to specialized provisions. As in the United Kingdom, these services were dependent on finances, but there were less regional variations within the country because the funding, whatever the amount, was far more centralized.

In Poland, there has been a long tradition of care for children with all forms of disabilities who have always enjoyed access to specialized services (Brykczynska, 1991). In some instances the care might have been seen as overly protectionist, but in the context of Central Europe, it is difficult to assess the extent to which this was overly patronizing and the extent to which it was a realistic necessity. Thus children did, and still do, attend special schools for the blind, deaf, physically disabled and such like. Mainstreaming is the exception rather than the rule. On the other hand many of the youngsters, in the spirit of Article 23, are prepared increasingly for meaningful work and life in the adult world. There are now quite effective self-help groups that speak for the concerns and needs of children and young adults with various disabilities. Perhaps the biggest problem area is in care for and co-operation with children with multiple handicaps and their families. With health care and social budgets ridiculously low, the care of this group of children is indeed inadequate and noticeably severely underfunded. Philip Darbyshire (1989), commenting on the Ten Whys (Whyns) of society and health care workers with regard to multiply handicapped children, could have been speaking of the prevailing attitude towards such children in Poland and in most of Central Europe (Figure 7.1).

This is not an unusual attitude, but where resources are low, equity and just allocation of resources seem to take low priority.

Indeed, as Darbyshire notes, it is not just a matter of resources, it is also a moral stance. To echo the Ten Whys (Whyns) sums up much of society's attitude towards these children. The resolution to the problem will have to come from an increased ethical awareness among social workers and nurses and others working with children.

The Polish Nurses' Association, with the help of moral philosophers and nurses, runs various workshops and seminars during the year on ethical issues in practice using the humanities to increase sensitivities. Additionally, senior child advocates, lawyers and politicians call for more understanding for this group of children. Hopefully, this will lead to a marked improvement in the way that these profoundly handicapped children are regarded and treated and hopefully, in the long term, they will be accorded those human rights to which they can lay legitimate claim. The children have a right to security, warmth, adequate food, nurture and where appropriate, as Article 23 notes, education and training that will help them achieve the greatest possible self-reliance and an active life, in a more considerate and morally responsive society.

Ten Whys (Whyns)

1. Why talk to them – they can't hear;
2. Why listen to them – they can't tell us anything;
3. Why ask them – they can't choose;
4. Why teach them – they can't learn;
5. Why show them – they can't see;
6. Why give them food – they can't taste any difference;
7. Why change them – they'll only wet and soil again;
8. Why give them toys – they can't play;
9. Why take them out – they don't notice anything;
10. Why bother ....?

(Darbyshire, 1989)

Figure 7.1   Darbyshire's Ten Whys (Whyns)

Article 39

> The state is obliged to ensure that child victims of armed conflicts, torture, neglect, maltreatment or exploitation receive appropriate treatment for their recovery and social integration.

This article of the Children's Convention is perhaps the most paradoxical, since it is often state-inflicted harm, in the form of torture and exploitation, that prompts the necessity to ensure that the child victims of state terror have 'appropriate treatment for their recovery and social integration'. Even if the government of countries or local councils are not to blame for harm inflicted on children, they often turn a blind eye to the illegal conduct of its citizens or appear powerless in the face of organized crime.

Amnesty International recently produced a booklet highlighting the plight of children around the world who are victims of armed conflict, torture, societal neglect, maltreatment or exploitation (Amnesty International, 1995). Some of the harm done to children is deliberate and callously targeted at this vulnerable group, for example recruiting children into prostitution, 'buying' kidneys from minors, enlisting boys into the army and so on. Some of the harm is aimed at children, because children represent a dispensable commodity. Exploitation of child labour, killing of street children in South America are prime examples. Finally, there is the harm done to children because they just happen to be in the way. Caught up in adult wars and the conflicts of adults, children, and often their mothers, become trapped in the middle, suffering physical, mental, psychological and spiritual damage. There are more orphaned and displaced children in Europe at this time than at any other since the conclusion of the Second World War. Although Western Europe is relatively free of state violence, bearing in mind that the children of Northern Ireland and the Basque region of Spain may disagree, Central Europe and the Russian Republic are experiencing ongoing massive social upheavals with resultant social chaos and lawlessness. The long drawn out war in the Balkans has resulted in a whole generation of youngsters becoming displaced witnesses of incredible violence and cruelty. Exploitation of children by organized crime, in the form of drug abuse, is prevalent in the whole of Europe and the recruitment of the street children of Moscow into organized criminal gangs by Mafia-style bandits is a growing problem. Closer to home, in the United Kingdom, the increase in homeless adolescents is of great concern, while the noticeable rise in child suicides and instances of serious bullying demonstrate the effects that societal stress and violence have on young impressionable individuals. The list of contemporary society's faults in respect of children is growing and the question is, 'to what extent is this of concern to health care workers generally and to paediatric nurses in particular, working in Europe?'

Certainly, the noticeable rise in the levels of stress and aggression in children is worrying and common throughout Europe. Children are appearing at schools, clinics and hospitals with stress-related disorders such as depression, anorexia, addictive behaviours, aggression and the like. Increasingly, children are acting out their fears and anxieties on each other, and the rise of serious death-inducing bullying in the United Kingdom is both distressing and alarming. The solutions to these problems will not be found by simply treating the children as passive recipients of 'bad luck', but as Amnesty International (1995) noted, by treating children 'as real people, like grown-ups (p. 1). The implication of this is that just as we would listen to the concerns, anxieties and fears of adults, so we should pay attention to the concerns of children. Under the terms of the Children's Convention, it is a child's right, not only to be 'rehabilitated', but also to expect to live through a 'childhood' free of exploitation and societal abuse. Signatories to the Convention need to look at what they are doing nationally to minimize harm and damage to children by adults. Harm of course is a loose concept and comes in a variety of forms. It might include physical punishment, which is still legal in the United Kindgom, trade in infants and young children as a response to the demand for adoptable children which is a huge problem in parts of southern Europe, or toleration of racial inequalities in health care provided to minority groups, a problem in much of Europe especially the United Kingdom, France and Germany.

Paediatric nurses are in a unique position to gain the trust of children and collectively to have a powerful voice which can demand change, as and when appropriate. The rights of children entail the duties of health workers involved in their care to stand up for the minimum securities needed to ensure an appropriate childhood for all children. The fact that for most European nurses their wages will be paid, directly or indirectly, by the state government, means that campaigning for social reforms to ease the fate of children may call for much courage and commitment on their part. This does not, however, absolve them from their responsibilities. In fact, as Amnesty International (1995) notes: 'Governments now have a duty, which many fail to carry out, to make the principles and provisions of the Convention widely known to adults and children alike' (p. 12).

Conclusion

Paediatric nurses all over Europe have a legal, as well as a moral, obligation to familiarize themselves with the content and spirit of the Children's Convention. Wherever possible they should work to implement the various articles and should join forces with other concerned adults to improve the lives of children.

From a concern for improved education of paediatric nurses across Europe to a united stand on physical punishment, child abuse or media exploitation of children, child health nurses have much to engage and occupy their social consciences. Perhaps the biggest change in paediatrics and the associated ethical issues in Europe over the last few years has been the realization that health concerns which affect children may have their roots outside of diseased and distressed bodies. In order to better answer the needs of children it has become necessary to approach the child in a broader, far more systematic, holistic fashion. Just as the political boundaries in Europe are coming down, so too are the Cartesian body–mind divisions of traditional approaches to health care. Shakespeare noted in *The Rape of Lucrece*, that 'if children pre-decease progenitors, we are their offspring, and they none of ours'. We must ensure the existence of a healthy generation of Europeans or we may find that our successors are unfit to survive us. Working towards ensuring that children's health rights are respected is one way that paediatric nurses can contribute to a future generation of healthy Europeans.

References

Ackerman, T.F. (1991) 'Innovative life saving treatments: do children have a moral right to receive them?', in Burgess, M.M. and Woodrow, B.E. (eds) *Contemporary Issues in Paediatric Ethics*. (The Edwin Mellen Press: Lewiston), pp. 41–56.

Alderson, P. (1990) *Choosing for Children: Parents' Consent to Surgery*. (Open University Press: Oxford).

Alderson, P. (1993) *Children's Consent to Surgery*. (Open University Press: Buckingham).

Almond, B. (1991) 'Rights', in Singer, P. (ed.) *A Companion to Ethics*. (Blackwell: Oxford), pp. 259–69.

Alston, P. (ed.) (1994) *The Best Interests of the Child: Reconciling Culture and Human Rights*. (Clarendon Press: Oxford).

Alston, P., Parker, S. and Seymour, J. (eds) (1992) *Children, Rights and the Law*. (Clarendon Press: Oxford).

Amnesty International (1995) *Childhood Stolen: Grave Human Rights Violations against Children*. (AI British Section: London).

Archard, D. (1993) *Children, Rights and Childhood*. (Routledge: London).

Beauchamp, T. and Childress, J. (1989) *Principles of Biomedical Ethics*, 3rd edn. (Oxford University Press: New York).

Beauchamp, T. and Childress, J. (1994) *Principles of Biomedical Ethics*, 4th edn. (Oxford University Press: New York).

Benjamin, M. and Curtis, J. (1992) *Ethics in Nursing*. (Oxford University Press: Oxford).

Brazier, M. and Lobjoit, M. (eds) (1991) *Protecting the Vulnerable: Autonomy and Consent in Health Care*. (Routledge: London).

Brykczynska, G. (ed.) (1989) *Ethics in Paediatric Nursing*. (Chapman & Hall: London).

Brykczynska, G. (1991) 'A Polish perspective', *Primary Health Care*, **1**(6): 20–1.

Brykczynska, G. (1993) 'Ethical issues in paediatric nursing', in Glasper, A. and Tuckee, A. *Advances in Child Health Nursing*. (Scutari Press: London), pp. 154–68.

Crawford, M. and Morris, M. (eds) (1994) *Neonatal Nursing*. (Chapman & Hall: London).

Darbyshire, P. (1989) 'Ethical issues in the care of the profoundly multiply-handicapped child', in Brykczynska, G. (ed.) *Ethics in Paediatric Nursing*. (Chapman & Hall: London), pp. 100–18.

Dimond, B. (1996) *The Legal Aspects of Child Health Care*. (Mosby: London).

Department of Health (1994) *The Clothier Report: The Allitt Inquiry*. (HMSO: London).

Edwards, J. (1996) 'Children with learning difficulties and the sacraments', *The Way Supplement 86: The Spirituality of Children*, 70–80.

Emson, H.E. (1992) 'Rights, duties and responsibilities in health care', *Journal of Applied Philosophy*, **9**(1): 3–11.

Fasting, U. (1995) 'The new iatrogenesis', in Lindrom, B. and Spencer, N. (eds) *Social Paediatrics*. (Oxford University Press: Oxford), pp. 259–69.

Hart, H.L.A. (1984 [1967]) 'Are there any natural rights?', in Waldron, J. *Theories of Rights*. (Oxford University Press: Oxford), pp. 77–90.

Hendrick, J. (1997) *Legal Aspects of Child Health Care*. (Chapman & Hall: London).

Kultgen, J. (1995) *Autonomy and Intervention*. (Oxford University Press: New York).

Leach, P. (1994) *Children First: What Society Must Do – and Is Not Doing for Children Today*. (Penguin: Harmondsworth).

Lifton, B.J. (1988) *The King of Children*. (Pan: London).

Long, I. (1992) 'To protect the public and ensure justice is done: an examination of the Philip Donnelly case', *Journal of Advanced Nursing*, **17**(1): 5–9.

Lumpp, Sr. Francesca (1982) 'Is health care a right?', in Curtin, L. and Flaherty, J. (eds) *Nursing Ethics: Theories and Pragmatics*. (Prentice-Hall: Englewood Cliffs, N.J.), pp. 25–33.

Matthews, G.B. (1994) *The Philosophy of Childhood*. (Harvard University Press: Cambridge, Mass.).

Montgomery, J. (1993) 'Consent to health care for children', *Journal of Child Law*, **5**(3): 1–8.

Newell, P. (1989) *Children are People Too: The Case against Physical Punishment*. (Bedford Square: London).

Newell, P. (1991) *The UN Convention and Children's Rights in the United Kingdom*. (National Children's Bureau: London).

Rawls, J. (1971) *A Theory of Justice*. (Harvard University Press: Cambridge, Mass.).

Reckling, J.B. (1994) 'Conceptual analysis of rights using a philosophic inquiry approach', *IMAGE: Journal of Nursing Scholarship*, **26**(4): 309–14.

Rogers, W.S. and Roche, J. (1994) *Children's Welfare and Children's Rights: A Practical Guide to the Law*. (Hodder & Stoughton, London).

Rosenbaum, M. and Newell, P. (1992) *Taking Children Seriously: A Proposal for a Children's Rights Commissioner*. (Calouste Gulbenkian Foundation: London).

Rubellin-Devichi, J. (1994) 'The best interests principle in French law and practice', in Altson, P. (ed.) *The Best Interests of the Child: Reconciling Culture and Human Rights*. (Clarendon Press: Oxford), pp. 259–80.

Slater, M. (1993) *Health for All Our Children: Achieving Appropriate Health Care for Black and Ethnic Minority Children and Their Families*. (Action for Sick Children: London).

Stainton, R.R., and Stainton, R.W. (1992) *Stories of Childhood: Shifting Agendas of Child Concern*. (Harvester Wheatsheaf: Hemel Hempstead).

UNCRC (The United Nations Committee of the Rights of the Child) (1995) 'Response to the UK report (1994) to UNCRC', reprinted in *Child Right*, 114, March, 3–5.

Upton, H. (1993) 'On applying moral theories', *Journal of Applied Philosophy*, **10**(2): 189–99.

Waldron, J. (1984) *Theories of Rights*. (Oxford University Press: Oxford).

Warnock, M. (1992) 'The nature of choice', in Warnock, M. (ed.) *Uses of Philosophy*. (Blackwell: Oxford), pp. 223–4.

Whyte, D.A. (1989) 'Ethics in neonatal nursing', in Brykczynska, G. (ed.) *Ethics in Paediatric Nursing*. (Chapman & Hall: London), pp. 23–41.

Worswick, J. (1993) *A House Called Helen: The Story of the First Hospice for Children*. (HarperCollins: London).

Suggestions for further reading

Emson, H.E. (1992) 'Rights, duties and responsibilities in health care', *Journal of Applied Philosophy*, **9**(1): 3–11.

Newell, P. (1991) *The UN Convention and Children's Rights in the United Kingdom*. (National Children's Bureau: London).

8

Ethical Issues in Integrating People with a Mental Handicap

Ruth Northway

Introduction

> It would be nice to say that so much time and effort does not need to be made just to allow people to be a part of the society in which they live. But it never really works out like that does it? (Souza with Ramcharan, 1997, p. 7).

Within every country in Europe there are people who are labelled as having a mental handicap. The word 'labelled' is used here deliberately as labels are seldom neutral. Moreover it draws attention to an important ethical dilemma which must be discussed, namely, which term should be used to refer to the group of people who form the focus of this chapter. This concern might be simply dismissed as a preoccupation with political correctness but the label which is applied to groups is one of the things which marks them out as 'different' and hence in need of integration.[1] As such, it is central to the debate within this chapter.

Terminology has varied throughout history and as one term becomes viewed as derogatory an alternative is advocated. At any one time, therefore, the choice of terms might vary both within and between countries. From the chapter title it can be seen that a decision to refer to this group as 'people with a mental handicap' has been taken. It is acknowledged that such terminology is viewed negatively by some people to whom the label is applied, preferring instead to be referred to as 'people with learning difficulties'. This preference is noted, respected and would be the preference of the author. However, as this volume is intended for a European audience, the use of 'people with a mental handicap' is defended on the basis that the term is the one which, at present, is most widely understood.

Once a group is perceived as 'different' this usually influences the manner in which they are treated by society. In the case of people who have a mental handicap their difference has often been viewed negatively, frequently resulting in their segregation[2] from wider society. This state of affairs is at last beginning to change and, throughout Europe, movement towards integration is being made. While this general trend can be observed, its implications inevitably vary from one country to another as a result of prevailing societal values, existing patterns of service provision and the economic resources that are available to effect change. Similarly, differences may be observed at both local and individual levels. Integration is therefore a complex process that requires both considerable time and effort (Souza with Ramcharan, 1997) and one which raises a number of ethical concerns.

Nurses, both specialist and generalist, have a role to play in this process. The exact nature of integration is closely dependent upon both the societal context in which it takes place and the social policies which promote or inhibit it. This chapter will discuss the nature of integration and provide an overview of the current situation in three European countries – Albania, the Republic of Ireland and the United Kingdom. Three broad aspects of integration which raise ethical concerns will be examined: the question of whether community living is a universal right; the issue of choice; and that of integration into health care systems. In each of these areas the implications for nursing practice will be considered. In conclusion, the key similarities and differences between the countries will be highlighted and the consequent challenges which face nurses and nursing identified.

The nature of integration

Meanings of integration

Integration means different things to different people. This is particularly true when adopting a European perspective as it may have different implications in each country. For the purposes of this chapter, however, it is necessary to arrive at a working definition.

The *Concise Oxford Dictionary* (Allen, 1991) defines integration as 'the intermixing of persons previously segregated' and to 'bring or come into equal membership of society'. Therefore, in relation to people who have a mental handicap, the movement towards integration involves not only a recognition that previously these people have not been viewed as part of society, but also a commitment to changing this situation. This is necessary as historically people who have a mental handicap have been segregated for a number of reasons, some of which might be viewed more positively than others. These include a lack of alternative facilities, the belief that specialist provision is the most appropriate form of support and societal prejudice.

Integration has gained momentum as a result of widespread acceptance of the principles of normalization which seek to promote 'an existence... as close to normal living conditions as possible' (Bank-Mikkelson, 1980, p. 56). Wolfensberger, one of the key proponents of normalization, suggested that integration was the opposite of segregation (Wolfensberger, 1972). He does, however, make a distinction between physical and social integration where the former means that people who have a mental handicap are in the physical presence of others. He makes this differentiation to stress the fact that mere physical presence, while it may promote social integration, does not in itself constitute full social integration which is the ultimate aim. Clearly then social integration has two components. As well as the use of community facilities it also involves relationships with others (Szivos, 1992). Integration therefore becomes a much broader issue than simply moving people out from segregated service provision.

Souza with Ramcharan (1997), speaking from personal experience of the 'separations' to which people who have a mental handicap may be subjected, discuss how, immediately a label is applied to children, they instantly become 'separated' from society as they are seen as different by their parents and others. This highlights one of the paradoxes involved in integration, as in order to change the situation, clear identification of those who have been segregated, and therefore need to be integrated, is necessary. However, this often involves the application of a 'label' which, while it identifies the group as requiring additional support, may have negative consequences as it further marks the group out as different and unfortunately, difference is often viewed negatively.

Integration is a concept which has been widely discussed at a European level and the European Union has since the 1980s had a programme which has sought to promote the integration of disabled people (the HELIOS programme). It is difficult, however, to speak of integration without placing it in a specific societal context as it is only by doing this that it is possible to determine its implications and hence the ethical issues which may arise. The current situation of people who have a mental handicap in three European countries, Albania, the Republic of Ireland and the United Kingdom, will therefore be examined.

Albania

Prior to the overthrow of the communist regime in March 1992, few details regarding life in Albania were known outside of the country. Swinburne (1994) provides some insight into the situation faced by people who have a mental handicap whose families were often ashamed to admit to their existence. As family support was virtually non-existent these people were left with the prospect of either coping alone or being sent to an institution. The location of institutions in the larger towns resulted in minimal family contact due to the distances involved and poor transport systems. Furthermore, conditions inside these children's homes were often poor; with bare rooms, little stimulation, staff who were not trained to meet the specific needs of the residents, heavy use of sedation and little emotional care (Swinburne, 1994). All of this suggests a very bleak picture and there is no reason to imagine that conditions for adults living in institutions were any better.

In theory, people in Albania who have a mental handicap have the same rights as other citizens. Educational law states that each mainstream class should be ready to accommodate at least two children who have a mild mental handicap and employment legislation states that every employer of more than 25 people should employ at least one disabled person. In practice these provisions are rarely enforced. As previously mentioned, one of the things which influences successful integration is the availability of economic resources to develop the necessary support systems. Similarly, integration has to take account of the prevailing societal conditions and attitudes at any given time. Both of these factors have had a significant impact on developments for people who have a mental handicap in Albania.

Things have begun to change since 1992 and, while there are still people with a mental handicap who find themselves in institutional provision, some progress has been made. Non-governmental organizations from within the country, such as the National Association for People with a Mental Handicap, along with external aid agencies such as the East European Partnership, have begun to work with the government to effect change. Specialist nurses and health professionals from other countries have been key members of these project teams.

As there was little societal understanding about the needs of people who have a mental handicap and those of their families (Swinburne, 1994), work to raise public awareness has been undertaken. In some areas support is being offered to families, projects to integrate children into mainstream classes have begun and some small group homes have been opened. Work is also under way in the institutions, although this has tended to focus on the provision of education and training for staff in an attempt to avoid the resentment caused by the provision of material aid, in a country where families are often so poor that they have difficulty in providing for their families' basic needs (Swinburne, 1994). Nurses are obviously key members of the staff teams within the institutions but, until recently, they were offered no specific training in relation to this client group. These educational developments have therefore increased both levels of understanding and the quality of care provision. Some restructuring of the institutions has also taken place.

Nurses also have a role to play outside of the institutions. For instance, health visitors provide advice and direct families to appropriate services, although this is obviously restricted by the limited services available. While progress has been made towards both integration and improving the quality of life for people who have a mental handicap within Albania, it has been slow and patchy. This is not meant to decry the progress that has been made, nor is it to argue that it should be halted. It does, however, illustrate how a legacy of underresourced services, together with a lack of societal awareness and restricted financial resources, limits the speed of change. It is perhaps significant that the project established by the East European Partnership, due to end in 1994 (Swinburne, 1994), is still operative in 1997. At the time of writing, Albania is once more in a period of civil unrest which has forced many foreign aid workers to leave and has prompted appeals for humanitarian aid. It is with some concern, therefore, that the situation of people with a mental handicap in Albania must be viewed.

The Republic of Ireland

The principle of community care for people who have a mental handicap has been broadly accepted within Ireland since the mid 1960s, although it was felt that community living would not be possible for everyone. A range of service provision was advocated which included accommodation within psychiatric hospitals, the development of smaller residential centres, some day services, educational provision and very limited family support. Present services are based primarily on the recommendations of the *Needs and Abilities* report (Review Group on Mental Handicap Services, 1990).

This document suggested that with the provision of appropriate services, the majority of people would be able to live in the community. While this may be seen as a statement of generally positive intent, it is important to note that it also raises the possibility that some people would not be able to live in the community and also that the ability of others to remain there is clearly linked to the availability of suitable support services. Nonetheless, it did advocate a number of key service developments, such as the need to ensure education for all children regardless of their disability, the need to provide a range of day, respite and other family support services and it also recognized the need for appropriately trained staff.

In relation to residential provision it was recommended that new residential centres should be as home-like as possible. The need to relocate those people who were inappropriately placed within psychiatric hospitals to more appropriate facilities was also identified as a priority. Placement in residential centres was identified as the 'least favoured option' except for certain groups of people (Review Group on Mental Handicap Services, 1990, Sect. 9: 5), including those with a severe or profound level of disability and those who have 'additional handicapping conditions'. The nature of these conditions, however, is not specified.

Progress towards these aims appears to be somewhat varied. Residential centres have become more home-like with the development of smaller living units. Although the level of funding has increased, enabling more residential places for emergency and respite care to be provided together with an expansion of home care provision, there is still a significant level of unmet need. For example, in 1994 there were said to be some 1300 people waiting for residential services and 1500 people waiting for day services (Department of Health, 1994).

The picture in relation to the accommodation of people who have a mental handicap within psychiatric hospitals is also unclear, even though their resettlement remains a priority (Department of Health, 1994). Estimates of the numbers of people involved vary between 942 in 1992 (Department of Health, 1994) to 1200 in 1996 (Commission on the Status of People with Disabilities, 1996). This may reflect both the difficulties and differences in classification, particularly of people who have a mild mental handicap. What is clear, however, is that a significant group of people continue to live in inappropriate and segregated settings. This is of particular concern when it is noted that the Commission on the Status of People with Disabilities (1996) found themselves to be 'greatly shocked by the poor standards of the physical accommodation' in some of these hospitals (Sect. 23: 18). While they recognized that financial constraints have been a major factor in inhibiting progress, there appears to be a gap between espoused policy and reality, and therefore the Commission called for the *Needs and Abilities* policy document to be reviewed as a matter of urgency.

Within Ireland there are specialist nurses for people who have a mental handicap (registered mental handicap nurses) working in a range of settings, such as hospitals, residential and day care centres, with people with varying degrees of disability and across all age groups. In addition, a small number of nurses are beginning to work directly with families in the home. Thus, specialist nurses are currently working in both segregated and integrated settings and appear to have a central role to play in promoting integration.

United Kingdom

While the majority of people who have a mental handicap have always lived in a community setting, the United Kingdom has a legacy of large-scale institutional provision. Official policy since the late 1950s has been to shift the focus of care from hospitals to community-based provision, but this has been a slow process. Prompted by concerns over conditions in the long-stay hospitals, the 1971 Government White Paper entitled *Better Services for the Mentally Handicapped* (Department of Health and Social Security, 1971) gave a renewed impetus to community integration. Its agenda for change involved both the improvement of conditions within existing institutions and the development of a range of community-based support services. In 1981 the Education Act made provision for children with special educational needs to be educated within mainstream educational provision. However, certain preconditions were set out before this could happen, namely that the education of the child should not suffer, the education of other children should not suffer and finally that it should make best use of available resources. Thus, while at one level there is a policy commitment to integration, a number of obstacles to its realization still exist.

In the mid 1990s a mixed picture has emerged. Current policy states that the priority is to support people to live in community settings through the development of an appropriate range of support services designed to complement existing patterns of family and community support. Some very good, innovative services exist, such as early support schemes, integrated placements within mainstream schools and supported employment schemes, but they are not available in all areas. Community-based services, for example day services, group homes, multidisciplinary community support teams and respite care services, have been developed, but again, there is a lack of uniformity and variations of both quantity and quality of service provision. Some long-stay institutions have been closed and many which remain have active resettlement programmes which are seeking to relocate residents into small-scale community living developments. It is likely that institutional care will remain part of service provision for a number of years and concerns have been expressed that the community services which have been developed are 'inadequate' (Cooke, 1997).

The United Kingdom has specialist nurses for people who have a mental handicap, although there has been an ongoing debate for a number of years as to whether such nurses are required. Interestingly, this debate has arisen partly because if the principles of normalization and integration are taken to their logical conclusion, then people who have a mental handicap would utilize ordinary community services, including health care facilities which employ generalist rather than specialist nurses (Cooke, 1997). Currently, specialist nurses work either in residential settings such as hospitals and small-scale group homes or in a domiciliary capacity, visiting families and clients who live independently or in group homes. Additionally, a number of qualified nurses are employed by social services or voluntary agencies in day and residential services. It would appear, however, that while many of them are employed because of their nursing experience they are not employed as nurses.

Ethical aspects of integration

From the preceding discussion it is evident that while there are variations between countries there are also similarities which will be of concern to nurses. Although it is clearly impossible to discuss all of these, some key areas will be explored.

A right to community living?

Stainton (1994) suggests that initial moves towards deinstitutionalization were primarily concerned with establishing the 'right form of care' rather than with concern for individual rights. Times have changed, however, and most services tend to view the concept of integration into 'normal community living' as a 'right' of people who have a mental handicap (Kay, 1994). Indeed, in this chapter it has been seen that in each of the countries, explicit policies exist which seem to support this goal to varying degrees. It has also been seen that gaps exist between policy and practice and that many people remain in segregated services. For nurses there appear to be three important areas to consider. First, the question of whether community living is a universal right. Second, the nature of the support required and lastly, the impact of the changes on conditions in any remaining segregated provision.

Kay (1994) argues that many of the assertions concerning the rights of people who have a mental handicap centre on the recognition of the personhood of the individual and as such involve moral rights rather than legal ones. It is interesting to note, therefore, that in Ireland admission to residential centres is viewed as the 'least favoured option' except for those who have severe or profound disabilities and those who have additional handicapping conditions (Review Group on Mental Handicap Services, 1990). Similarly, in the UK these are the groups who have often been the last to be considered for resettlement from hospitals and for whom some form of continuing health care provision is often thought necessary. This seems to suggest that some groups of people are viewed as having less of a right to live in a community setting than others. As it is these groups with whom nurses most often work, the issues involved require further examination.

It has often been argued that the level of need for people who have a severe or profound mental handicap can only be met within an institutional setting. This has been challenged by Tossebro *et al*. (1996) who stated that the necessity for institutions began to be questioned in Scandinavia in the 1980s and, while it was accepted that these people needed a high level of support, the link between this need and institutional care can be broken. What is vital in this debate is that the rights of people with multiple and profound disabilities to live in a community setting are not advocated at the expense of ensuring that both the individual and his or her family have the appropriate range of support services available. Clearly, it is possible for people living in the community to remain isolated because of unmet needs for support. However, it is also essential that a lack of services is not used as an excuse to limit the extent to which a group of people are integrated. That is to argue, as has happened in the past, that they 'need' institutions. The issue seems to be one of resource availability, rather than the ability of the individual who has a mental handicap, and nurses may find themselves placed in the position of advocate for their patient or client. The extent to which nurses can perform this function may be limited by the fact that they are often employed by the agency providing the services, and therefore the nurse may need to ensure that the client has access to an independent advocate.

A further group of people whose rights to live in a community setting are often questioned are those whose behaviour challenges. One widely quoted definition of challenging behaviour, as well as that referring to behaviour which may harm the individual or others, refers to behaviours which may limit or deny access to ordinary community facilities (Blunden and Allen, 1987). The extent to which a behaviour segregates or threatens to segregate an individual is, therefore, one of the key factors in defining whether or not the behaviour challenges.

Kay (1994) argues that if people have a right to live in the community they also have an obligation to behave in a manner which is in keeping with societal expectations. Clearly there are some behaviours which cannot be tolerated such as extreme physical violence. In such cases it may be necessary to provide some form of intensive support service for a specific period of time. Such examples are rare, however, and on a day-to-day basis the nurse is more likely to be concerned with clients whose behaviour, although it does no physical harm, may serve to segregate them from wider society. The focus of concern therefore should be on what constitutes acceptable behaviour and who decides this (Kay, 1994). Should the nurse ensure that individuals acquire socially acceptable behaviours or should society be expected to be more tolerant? Clearly, in the short term, society is unlikely to change and therefore the reality is that people who have a mental handicap will continue to be excluded if they do not conform to the prevailing standards (Cooke, 1997). Consequently, the nurse has to work with individuals to determine which is the most appropriate course of action for them. There is also an important role for nurses in raising public awareness of the needs of people who have a mental handicap and the importance of this has been recognized in Albania. While this may be a long-term strategy, it may increase understanding and perhaps lead to greater tolerance of individual differences.

The above examples highlight the role of support services in realizing the integration of people who have a mental handicap. In Albania it was noted that many parents had no option but to admit their child to institutional care because of the lack of community-based services (Swinburne, 1994). Such a scenario is not confined to Albania, however. In Britain, institutional closure has resulted in 'inadequate provision for many and no service for some' (Cooke, 1997) and, in Ireland, it is not clear how many people on the waiting list for residential care could be supported in the community if adequate services were available (Department of Health, 1994). Nurses working in community settings are an important part of such support services both in terms of the direct service which they offer and the co-ordinating function which they perform. If institutional care is to be reduced, an adequate range of community-based services are required, both to alleviate the need for admission to residential care and to promote integration.

This highlights a further area of potential concern. The analysis of the current situation in each of the three European countries has identified that, along with public attitudes, one of the major factors inhibiting progress towards integration is the limited availability of financial resources. The essential question which arises relates to where resources can be used to best effect. One possible solution is for money to be spent only on new developments rather than on improving existing segregated provision. This, however, raises ethical concerns for nurses who, as the main care providers in these segregated residential settings, have a concern for the quality of life of the people they support.

It has been seen that while some improvements have been made in standards of care, concerns about the physical conditions within psychiatric hospitals in Ireland (Commission on the Status of People with Disabilities, 1996) and in institutions in Albania (Swinburne, 1994) have been expressed. Similarly, in the United Kingdom, moves towards integration were prompted by anxieties about the quality of institutional care. Nurses appear to be in a difficult position here, as by arguing for the improvement of institutions, they may be criticized for seeking to defend their continued employment. However, tolerating poor physical conditions for their patients and clients could also leave nurses open to criticisms of neglect. Clearly, nurses must be accountable for their actions and the consequences of their decisions and they must be prepared to defend their judgement (Kay, 1994).

Choice

The decision to move away from segregated forms of service provision is usually one that is based, in part, on financial considerations but also on the belief that such a move would improve the quality of life for people who have a mental handicap. Although this line of reasoning is accepted by many people, inevitably there will be individuals who feel that such a view is not right for them and is paternalistic.

Wolfensberger (1972) argues that devaluation is compounded when people who are devalued by society mix with other people who are similarly devalued. He suggests instead, that if these people wish to avoid devaluation, they should associate with valued people and shun the company of devalued people. Such a position ignores the benefits which some people may derive from such associations and there is a danger that, in accepting such a philosophy, integration will be imposed rather than chosen. This could raise some dilemmas for nurses working in a system which seeks to promote integration with individuals who do not wish to integrate.

Disregarding the views of people who have a mental handicap about their day-to-day lives might be viewed as treating them as 'less than human' (Chadwick and Tadd, 1992, p. 128). However, it could also be argued that if there is a policy of integration, then the individual has no real choice in the matter. Indeed while most people expect to be offered some choice, a completely free choice is seldom offered as options are limited by a lack of goods, time or resources (Cooke, 1997). In this instance there is a clash between a policy which is believed to be of benefit to a group of people and the wishes of the individual. This represents a clash between the moral principle of beneficence and that of autonomy. In relation to people who have a mental handicap this is further complicated by the fact that they are frequently not viewed as being capable of autonomous decision-making (Chadwick and Tadd, 1992). Moreover, a lack of competence in one area of life is often taken as inferring generalized incompetence (Brown *et al.*, 1992). The challenge for nurses therefore, is to facilitate informed decision-making wherever this is possible. This means that nurses need to work with individuals, to develop decision-making skills, to enable them to clarify the extent of their options and identify the possible consequences of the various courses of action, as well as to support them in their decisions.

Integration into health care

The sections discussed above might be viewed simply as representing the concerns of specialist nurses who work solely with people who have a mental handicap. However, if people who have a mental handicap are to be integrated into society, it follows that they will need to be integrated into the existing health care systems to ensure that their health needs are met.

The integration of people who have a mental handicap therefore becomes the concern of every nurse.

All people who have a mental handicap have the same health needs as the rest of the population, although these are sometimes obscured by their disability. Some, however, have additional health needs as a result of their underlying impairment (Welsh Health Planning Forum, 1992). If these needs are not met, additional restrictions are imposed on the individual, compounding their underlying impairment and limiting the possibilities for their integration. It is essential, therefore, that people who have a mental handicap have access to health care.

In each of the countries chosen for discussion, people with a mental handicap theoretically have the same rights of access to health care as other citizens in their respective countries. In Ireland there is a policy commitment which states that they have the same rights of access to government services as other citizens (Review Group on Mental Handicap Services, 1990). In the United Kingdom it is stated that:

> People with learning disabilities (mental handicap) have the same rights of access to National Health Service services as everyone else (National Health Service Executive, 1992, p. 1).

However, simply stating that people have equal access does not take account of their varying needs and may result in unequal outcomes. The National Health Service Executive (NHSE, 1992) recognizes that people who have a mental handicap may require additional assistance to use health services. As Kay (1994) suggests, 'if justice means that unequals should be treated unequally then someone needs to be concerned with the unequals' (p. 87).

There would appear to be a gap between policy and practice. In gathering the information for this chapter, one area of concern common to each of the countries was the difficulties in accessing health care which people who have a mental handicap experience. There may be a number of reasons as to why this is the case, such as communication difficulties on the part of both health professionals and the person with a mental handicap, inadequate training and support of carers and societal prejudice. While each of these has implications for nurses, it is the latter which perhaps raises specific ethical concerns.

Where resources for health care are limited, then health services tend to be targeted or rationed. This raises particular concerns in relation to people who have a mental handicap, as they may be excluded from health care by virtue of their disability. The issue at stake here is that of respect for person-hood, for if we argue that all people by virtue of being human have a right to be valued, then it follows that they also have an equal right to appropriate treatment.

Nurses and other health care professionals are members of society and as such, may have the same prejudices towards people who have a mental handicap. A key factor in promoting better access to health care for people who have a mental handicap is, therefore, the improvement of nursing education. In Albania, training is being provided by non-governmental organizations and within the UK, all student nurses undertake theoretical and practical experience in relation to people who have a mental handicap within the Common Foundation Programme. Similarly, in Ireland, there are calls for disability awareness training to be provided for all health service staff (Commission on the Status of Disabled People, 1996). While awareness may be an important and necessary first step, it is important that it is translated into positive action. This needs to include action at both the level of individual practice and at service and policy levels to ensure that the health system is receptive and responsive to the needs of people who have a mental handicap. Nurses have a role to play at all levels.

Conclusion

Each of the countries examined in this chapter is seeking to promote the integration of people who have a mental handicap and, while much remains to be done, some progress is evident. In each country nurses play a major role in this process. While variations, due largely to differing historical legacies and the level of resources available to effect change, are apparent, some common areas of concern have also emerged between the countries.

One central issue is the question of choice. In each of the countries people have been admitted to institutional care as a result of inadequate community-based services. There was no choice. Similarly, there are those clients who may prefer not to integrate, but find themselves in a situation where policy dictates that this is not an option. The challenge is therefore to provide a range of services capable of meeting both the needs and preferences of individuals, while recognizing that these needs and preferences may change over time.

Another common theme that has emerged is the role played by economic support in bringing about change. Difficulties exist in each country and just as the nature and extent of these problems vary, so too does the impact on nursing practice. There is a difficult balance to be struck between ensuring that appropriate community-based facilities are developed before institutions close, while at the same time ensuring that material conditions within institutions do not deteriorate to unacceptably low standards. As nurses work in both institutional and community settings they may find themselves at the centre of such debates, and inevitably this will impinge on their practice.

A particularly disturbing commonality between countries, which surfaced while researching and writing this chapter, is the difficulty which people who have a mental handicap face when seeking access to health care. Consequently, all nurses must examine their practice in this area, as a matter of urgency, if the situation is to improve.

One overarching challenge is the need for nurses to work at a variety of levels. The importance of working with the individual to ensure that his or her needs and wishes are taken into account has been highlighted. However, by definition, integration means that the individual has to be integrated 'into' something. What this means for nurses is that, although their primary focus may be on their patient or client, they cannot disregard the other part of the equation, namely society. Indeed, a number of the ethical issues which have been highlighted will not be resolved simply by working with the individual. Nurses must have a thorough awareness of the communities and societies in which they work, of the social policies which shape them and of how power operates within them. In short they must be politically aware.

It is not possible in a chapter of this length to explore all of the ethical issues which can arise for nurses when seeking to promote the integration of people who have a mental handicap. This is particularly true as the exact implications will vary from country to country and from individual to individual. However, as Kay (1994) suggests, one of the problems which we face when we encounter ethical dilemmas is finding a 'way in'. It is hoped that, in examining some common dilemmas, this chapter will promote discussion between nurses, helping them to find a 'way in', and thereby contribute to the provision of more positive support for people who have a mental handicap, regardless of where they live.

Notes

1. The process through which people with a mental handicap become recognized as full members of society. Integration may be physical, whereby they are physically part of their community, or social, whereby social relationships are developed.
2. The process through which people with a mental handicap become separated from wider society. This may be physical, for example in specialist services, and/or social, when they are subjected to negative discriminatory attitudes.

References

Allen, R.E. (1991) *The Concise Oxford Dictionary of Current English*, 8th edn. (Oxford University Press: Oxford).

Bank-Mikkelson, N. (1980) 'Denmark', in Flynn, R.J. and Nitsch, K.E. (eds) *Normalisation, Social Integration and Community Services*. (Pro-Ed: Austin, Tex.), pp. 50–71.

Blunden, R. and Allen, D. (1987) *Facing the Challenge: An Ordinary Life for People with Learning Difficulties and Challenging Behaviour*. (King's Fund: London).

Brown, J.M., Kitson, A.L. and McKnight, T.J. (1992) *Challenges in Caring: Explorations in Nursing and Ethics*. (Chapman & Hall: London).

Chadwick, R. and Tadd, W. (1992) *Ethics and Nursing Practice: A Case Study Approach*. (Macmillan: Basingstoke).

Commission on the Status of People with Disabilities (1996) *A Strategy for Equality*. (The Stationery Office: Dublin).

Cooke, P. (1997) 'Learning disability', in Skidmore, D. (ed.) *Community Care: Initial Training and Beyond.* (Arnold: London), pp. 237–57.

Department of Health (1994) *Shaping a Healthier Future: A Strategy for Effective Health Care in the 1990s.* (The Stationery Office: Dublin).

Department of Health and Social Security (1971) *Better Services for the Mentally Handicapped.* Cmnd 4683. (HMSO: London).

Kay, B. (1994) 'People with learning difficulties', in Tschudin, V. (ed.) *Ethics: Nursing People with Special Needs.* (Scutari Press: London), pp. 1–43.

National Health Service Executive (1992) *Health Services for People with Learning Disabilities (Mental Handicap)*, Health Service Guidelines (92)42. (Department of Health: London).

Review Group on Mental Handicap Services (1990) *Needs and Abilities: A Policy for the Intellectually Disabled.* (The Stationery Office: Dublin).

Souza, A. with Ramcharan, P. (1997) 'Everything you ever wanted to know about Down's Syndrome but never bothered to ask', in Ramcharan, P., Roberts, G., Grant, G. and Borland, J. (eds) *Empowerment in Everyday Life: Learning Disability.* (Jessica Kingsley: London), pp. 3–14.

Stainton, T. (1994) *Autonomy and Social Policy.* (Avebury: Aldershot).

Swinburne, S. (1994) 'New society', *Nursing Times*, **90**(29): 48–9.

Szivos, S. (1992) 'The limits to integration?', in Brown, H. and Smith, H. (eds) *Normalisation: A Reader for the Nineties.* (Routledge: London), pp. 112–33.

Tossebro, J., Aalto, M. and Brusen, P. (1996) 'Changing ideologies and patterns of services: the Nordic countries', in Tossebro, J., Gustavsson, A. and Dyrendahl, G. (eds) *Intellectual Disabilities in the Nordic Welfare States.* (HoyskoleForlaget: Kristiansand), pp. 45–66.

Welsh Health Planning Forum (1992) *Protocol for Investment in Health Gain: Mental Handicap (Learning Disabilities).* (Welsh Office: Cardiff).

Wolfensberger, W. (1972) *The Principle of Normalisation in Human Services.* (National Institute on Mental Retardation: Toronto).

Suggestions for further reading

Coupe, J., O'Kane, J. and Golbart, J. (eds) (1996) *Whose Choice?: Contentious Issues for Those Working with People with Learning Difficulties.* (David Fulton: London).

Gates, B. and Beacock, C. (eds) (1997) *Dimensions of Learning Disability.* (Baillière Tindall: London).

Hutchison, P. and McGill J. (1992) *Leisure, Integration and Community.* (Leisureability: Ontario).

Mental Health Foundation Committee of Inquiry (1996) *Building Expectations: Opportunities and Services for People with a Learning Disability.* (The Mental Health Foundation: London).

Northway, R. (1997) 'Integration and inclusion: illusion or progress in services for disabled people', *Social Policy and Administration*, **31**(2): 157–72.

9

Ethical Issues in Mental Health Nursing

Kevin Gournay

Introduction

Mental health problems are so common that at some point in our lives all of us will be affected either by personal experience or the experience of those close to us. Thus, for example, the lifetime prevalence of schizophrenia, the most severe and enduring of mental illness, is 1 per cent and of depression more than 20 per cent (Department of Health, 1994). We know that roughly one in three of us will have a panic attack or panic attacks during our lifetime (Gournay, 1996) and up to 40 per cent of all general practitioner (GP) consultations concern medical problems for which no physical cause is evident. Mental health problems range from discrete episodes of anxiety and depression which last no more than a few days, to the most serious and enduring forms of illness such as schizophrenia and bipolar affective disorder. There is no simple spectrum covering the positions between these two extremes; mental health problems are best conceptualized as being multifaceted and multidimensional. Problems often present themselves somewhat paradoxically. For example, people with the most severe obsessions and compulsions may spend literally hours a day washing their hands while at the same time lead a very productive life in one of the professions and also have major familial and parental responsibilities. Similarly, victims of bipolar affective illness, more commonly known as manic depression, may have periods when they are unable to make any rational decisions and may need to be detained in hospital against their will. However, in between episodes of illness, this person may occupy a position of great responsibility in society.

The nature of mental health nursing reflects the above complexity of mental health problems and the practice of this branch of nursing cannot be easily defined. While mental health problems have remarkably similar incidences throughout both the developed and underdeveloped world, the disparate views of mental illness held by various cultures have led to great differences in approaches to care and treatment. As we will see below, in Europe at least, there are a number of common characteristics of mental health services present in many countries. For example, the care of the mentally ill is now firmly located within the community in many (though not all) Western countries and institutional facilities are, to a large extent, being closed.

The most radical deinstitutionalization policies were enacted in Italy in the 1970s (Battaglia, 1987). However, although there was a great upheaval in services at the time of the legislation, the country now boasts some exemplary initiatives. These include work co-operatives for the mentally ill and a number of innovative accommodation programmes (Mosher and Burti, 1994). In the Netherlands, people with a serious and enduring mental illness are often 'fostered' within the community and such schemes have undoubtedly helped to reduce the stigma associated with such problems (Decker *et al.*, 1995).

Throughout Europe, many mental health nurses are increasingly required to adopt new roles in the community which are very dissimilar from those previously occupied in hospital settings. However, service provisions are by no means homogeneous either across Europe or even within countries. Recently a national research project carried out by the Clinical Standards Advisory Group of the United Kingdom (Department of Health, 1995) showed a great diversity of service provision and quality of care across the four home countries.

This chapter can only provide a starting-point for thinking about the ethics of mental health and mental health nursing. In order to provide context, some of the different nursing roles are described in more detail. Following that, a review will be undertaken of a number of areas of particular importance to mental health nurses which should together provide a basis for considering ethical issues in theory and practice. As previously mentioned, there are a number of similarities among services across Europe and the areas chosen for consideration are those which are most commonly found in many European countries.

Overview of mental health provision in Europe

In order to understand some of the issues connected with the ethical aspects of mental health nursing, it is important to understand the context. Unlike other forms of nursing, mental health nursing need not be completely located within the health sector. In the United Kingdom most mental health nurses are employed either within the National Health Service or increasingly, within the private sector – either in private hospitals or nursing homes. However, in other parts of Europe the situation is different. In the Netherlands, for example, mental health care in the community is largely located within 'not for profit' foundations which combine health, social services and other personnel, with local government providing some facilitative functions. Italy, on the other hand, has placed greater emphasis on the social aspects of mental health care and the country has a network of social care co-operatives. Many countries are now deriving funding for health services from insurance schemes and within these systems care is more medically, rather than socially, dominated. These insurance schemes may be private, as in the UK where the percentage of the population with private cover is rising each year. Or they may be a mixture of state-funded and private schemes, as found in Germany. Although the level of cover provided varies considerably, it is rare for continuing or long-term mental health problems to be covered by health insurance.

The deinstitutionalization referred to above is a complex and extremely variable phenomenon. The greatest decline in bed numbers has taken place in Italy and the United Kingdom, while the numbers of people in hospital beds in France, the Netherlands and Greece has declined at a much slower rate.

Another principle which is important to consider in understanding how services are being delivered and how ethical thinking may be formed is that of normalization. As Ramon (1996) notes, normalization is a much clearer concept than community care, as it focuses on the rights of people with any kind of disability to an ordinary life; on the provision of opportunities for such a life; and the removal of material and attitudinal obstacles to it. Ramon also notes that normalization has become a much more important issue in the UK, Italy and Scandinavia than in the countries of southern, Central or Eastern Europe. As we shall see below when considering the issue of treatment against the person's wishes, the importance of considering the perspective of service users in treatment decisions is crucial. The reader should therefore bear in mind that in some European countries normalization is not a principle which applies to mental health care. In these countries, therefore, the issue of giving patients treatment against their will is obviously viewed in a very different manner than it is in those countries in which a more liberal atmosphere maintains.

The nature of mental health nursing

Despite deinstitutionalization, mental health nurses work in hospitals, of both the large asylum type and in smaller psychiatric units in district general hospitals. Increasingly, however, they also work in various community settings including patients' homes. Nurses working in hospital settings have functions which are in many ways similar to their general nursing colleagues. Treatment in these settings is clearly prescribed by the responsible medical officer and nursing tasks are usually fairly well defined. Nurses are responsible for giving medication, running therapeutic groups and observing patients. Nurses are responsible for planning programmes of nursing care for in-patients, but there are clear definitions of the areas of responsibility. In community settings, these responsibilities are much less clear. For example, community psychiatric nurses may function in a number of different ways. At one end of the spectrum they may, like their hospital counterparts, have clearly defined roles, such as the giving of medication and the monitoring of symptoms. Indeed, this was the original basis on which the first community psychiatric nursing service in England started from Warlingham Park Hospital in 1954 (Moore, 1961). Currently, community psychiatric nurses are taking on a wider range of responsibilities and are often designated as the key worker.

In the United Kingdom, key worker responsibilities are presently defined within a legal framework, that is, the Care Programme Approach (Department of Health, 1989). Such responsibilities confer greater autonomy on the nurse, in the sense of more powers of decision-making and a wider brief for implementing a number of interventions without deferral to a psychiatrist. Not all key workers are nurses, however, and a recent national review, commissioned by the Sainsbury Centre for mental health and chaired by Rabbi Julia Neuberger (1997), has recognized that mental health nursing roles overlap considerably with those of other professions.

This review has noted that the case manager or key worker role for people with a serious mental illness being cared for and treated in the community may be undertaken by any mental health professional or indeed non-professional. To emphasize this point, Filson and Kendrick (1997) recently reported a considerable overlap in the roles of occupational therapists and nurses working in the community. In the United Kingdom, key workers in the community usually come from a nursing background, while in the United States, such key workers usually come from a social work background. In Europe, case manager roles are increasingly developing, although the level of responsibility and autonomy given to key workers varies tremendously, not only between countries but also within them. Case management models, such as the one in Verona in Italy, have been common in European countries for many years and these are now being applied in former Eastern bloc countries such as the Czech Republic (Pfeiffer, 1993). As previously mentioned, these case managers may have a greater level of autonomy with considerable responsibility for organizing and delivering treatment programmes. Thus, with this responsibility comes a need to be aware of the ethical issues.

In many countries mental health nurses have developed very specific psychotherapeutic roles. The first preparatory training programmes in behavioural psychotherapy were established at the Maudsley Hospital in London in 1972 to enable nurses to undertake this element of care (Marks *et al.*, 1977; Marks, 1985). These programmes explicitly set out to train nurses as autonomous therapists in a range of anxiety disorders such as agoraphobia and obsessive compulsive disorder and as therapists for common sexual conditions, such as premature ejaculation, anorgasmia and vaginismus. More controversially, nurse therapists were trained to deliver the treatment of sexual problems where the behaviour can be viewed as 'abnormal', for example, exhibitionism, paedophilia and fetishism. These nursing roles are now commonplace in some parts of Europe, for example in the Netherlands and Scandinavia, and training in these therapeutic techniques is now beginning in former Eastern bloc countries such as the Czech Republic.

A recent and similar nurse educational development in the treatment and management of serious mental illness is that of the Thorn Initiative (Lancashire *et al.*, 1997). Although this programme was originally designed for nurses, it is now open to other mental health professionals, including psychologists, social workers and occupational therapists. The aim of the Thorn programme is to train case managers working in community settings in an array of research-based treatment techniques appropriate for people with schizophrenia. These include: cognitive behavioural interventions for psychotic symptoms; the use of family management techniques emphasizing family stress management and problem-solving; as well as a range of skills connected with case management. This programme is currently only available in the UK, although there are similar, but less extensive, training programmes in Australia (O'Halloran *et al.*, 1995). Within a few years, however, it is likely that similar programmes of training will be established in Scandinavia and the Republic of Ireland.

It is evident, then, that mental health nurses may work in a variety of settings, with people who are experiencing a wide spectrum of mental health problems, for which a wide range of interventions can be used. In addition, mental health nurses have acquired various levels of autonomy. There is no simple way of examining all of the ethical dilemmas faced by nurses within the limits of a single chapter and therefore, in order to capture many of the issues involved, five key areas have been selected. These have been chosen as they represent some of the most difficult problems encountered by mental health nurses in trying to balance the interests of people with mental health problems with those of the wider society. Also, these issues reflect the vulnerability of this client group. They are:

- Confidentiality
- Sexual and personal relationships
- Treatment against the patient's will and the use of legal measures
- Continuing professional development
- Issues connected with the elderly with mental health problems.

Confidentiality

Mental health nurses face particular problems in connection with this aspect of their practice. Clause 10 of the UKCC's *Code of Professional Conduct* (1992) requires nurses to 'keep confidential any information obtained during the course of professional practice and to make disclosures only with the consent, where required, by the order of a court, albeit she/he can justify disclosure in the wider public interest'. On one hand, when the nurse is acting as a therapist, for example treating someone who suffers a very intimate sexual difficulty, there is both an implicit and explicit understanding that whatever the patient discloses to the nurse is in the strictest confidence. However, in other circumstances, nurses have a duty to disclose certain information to professional colleagues, carers or others. In these cases it can be argued that such disclosure is necessary for the patient's care or to protect the patient or others from possible harm.

Let us examine some of these issues. First, nurses often look after people with serious and enduring mental illnesses such as schizophrenia. As a consequence of that illness, a person may develop a wish or plan to commit an act of violence. While we know that the media portrayal of the seriously mentally ill as violent is generally unfair, there is no doubt that rates of violence among the seriously mentally ill are higher than those found among the general population and such phenomena are common enough to affect most community nurses. Indeed this problem has achieved formal recognition in the establishment, by the Department of Health, of the Confidential Inquiry into Homicides by People with a Mental Illness. There are, of course, notable examples of violence by mentally ill people and perhaps the most widely reported case was that of Christopher Clunis who stabbed a complete stranger, Jonathan Zito, to death on Finsbury Park tube station in December 1992. The subsequent inquiry (Ritchie *et al.*, 1994) showed that Christopher Clunis's care was very poorly co-ordinated and that communication between all the agencies involved in his case, namely the police, social workers, psychiatrists and nurses, failed repeatedly. One of the key issues in this failure of communication was that of workers in the various agencies not reporting to others, information which suggested that Christopher Clunis had a propensity to cause serious harm. In such cases, nurses have a clear duty to disclose information which they may have obtained within the context of their professional relationship so as to prevent harm befalling members of the general public. To whom then should this information be transmitted? Clearly there is a duty to convey this information to all other members of the multidisciplinary team. However, in many cases there may be grounds for reporting such information to the police. Many European countries are now following the example set by Scandinavian countries and are developing police/mental health services liaison schemes to deal with such difficulties. Italy has a number of these schemes in place, as does the United Kingdom.

Liaison schemes facilitate co-operation with the police and help to ensure that the patient's problems are dealt with as sensitively as possible. Mental health services across Europe are all developing more sophisticated information systems so that care can be properly co-ordinated. However, there is also a world-wide trend towards specifically identifying patients who are at particular risk of harming themselves or others by using mechanisms such as supervision registers. Without doubt, there will be many cases where disclosure of information to the police is very reasonable, as the central reason for disclosure is the protection of the public. Normally, if the nurse feels that there is a danger of the patient coming to some harm or harming others, this information should be shared with the psychiatrist who bears the ultimate responsibility for the patient's care and treatment. In some circumstances, however, as in the case of community psychiatric nurses working 'on call' duties at night, the nurse may have to exercise discretion and contact the police immediately. Wherever possible, such disclosure should be the responsibility of the psychiatrist in charge.

Gradually, mental health services have begun to recognize that working with people with serious and enduring illnesses poses problems concerning confidentiality and increasingly staff are guided by a range of locally developed policies. The nurse has a moral, as well as a professional, duty to understand these policies before embarking on any autonomous actions. As a corollary of this, nurses are becoming increasingly aware of the need to have good clinical supervisory frameworks in place so that ethical and clinical problems can be discussed with a supervisor. In mental health services, this supervisor need not necessarily be a nurse and in many, a multidisciplinary supervision model is employed, with one specific individual acting as a facilitator. Any breach of confidentiality is serious and striking a balance between maintaining patient trust and safeguarding the public's interest is one of the most difficult issues faced by mental health nurses.

Confidentiality in child sexual abuse

As highlighted in Chapter 7, concern about the sexual abuse of children is rising across Europe. Mental health nurses often work with children who may have experienced sexual abuse, and during the course of their work nurses may not only become aware of continuing abusive practices but also be in a position to identify the perpetrators of such actions. In England, the Children Act 1989, and the associated guideline Working Together under the Children Act 1989 (1991) make it clear that the prime responsibility of the worker is towards the interests of the children involved. The guideline emphasizes that if a worker becomes concerned that a child is being abused, then that worker needs to share that concern with other professionals in the team. This sharing of concern may of course involve breaking confidentiality with the child concerned so as to ensure that the abuse is brought to an end. In the case of children, the potential loss of trust that the child may experience is an extremely serious concern which must be carefully balanced.

As an extension of this problem, nurses may find themselves working with someone who is a perpetrator of sexual abuse, a situation which is most likely to confront nurses working as behaviour therapists who are specifically trained to treat such sexual problems. What happens, for example, if a paedophile is referred for treatment by a nurse therapist and then, during the course of treatment, the paedophile discloses that he has once again commenced paedophilic activity? There is no specific guidance based on any nursing codes of conduct which can be used by such nurses. However, the professional practice guidelines of the British Psychological Society for Clinical Psychologists (1995, p. 33) do provide some guidance for psychologists, although these materials stop short of giving clear, unequivocal advice. For example, the guidelines cite the following: 'a particular example of this balance of risk might involve the disclosure of a perpetrator of prior sexual abuse who is currently in contact with children, against the strong wishes of an adult survivor who is in therapy. There are no statutory requirements for psychologists to disclose in such situations.'

In summary, therefore, mental health nurses are faced with a range of very difficult situations involving confidentiality and the disclosure of information. Although there are several mechanisms for assisting nurses, such as locally developed guidelines and legal mechanisms, nurses must ensure that they use the multidisciplinary team to share particular problems and that they are able to access appropriate expertise for the purpose of clinical supervision.

Sexual and personal relationships

Although at first sight this seems to be a clearly defined area, it is one where there are potentially a number of problems for nurses. There is no doubt that at one end of the spectrum the issues are unambiguous. For example, in the United Kingdom it is a criminal act for a nurse to enter into a sexual relationship with a patient who is receiving in-patient psychiatric treatment. Similarly, a community nurse who is caring for a patient with a serious and enduring mental illness and who is, by definition, vulnerable, would be in clear breach of the professional code of conduct if he or she commenced a sexual relationship with that person. Suspicion that such acts are taking place may cause difficulties, however, for other members of the team. For example, all mental health nurses working in hospital settings will have experienced patients who make false claims against members of staff, for reasons connected with their mental illness. Such cases may include patients with paranoid illnesses who may claim, *inter alia*, that a member of staff is poisoning them, is in love with them and so on. Although such allegations may be made either maliciously or as part of the patient's illness, every allegation concerning possible abuse must be treated very seriously.

The central principle in such cases is that, unless there is an extremely good reason, allegations must be investigated properly. This must involve informing the police so that the matter may be investigated thoroughly and independently. It may be that information comes to light which suggests that abuse may have occurred, but the patient does not wish to make a complaint. In this case, there is still an obligation to investigate the matter properly, although considerable sensitivity will be needed by mental health staff and the police. Patients who have experienced sexual abuse by a member of staff may be reluctant to complain because they fear that the complaint will interfere with their treatment or, in some cases, the abusing member of staff may have used threats to ensure silence. In such cases, nursing staff must be prepared to act as an advocate for the patient. From an ethical standpoint, the nurse needs to keep in sharp focus that protection of the patient is paramount and all other considerations, in a sense, become secondary.

In recognition of these problems, many countries are becoming much more aware of the need to provide gender-sensitive intervention. Italy is perhaps the best example of innovation. For example, the Trieste mental health services now operate a service which focuses specifically on women and this service is provided by women mental health professionals. For more detail, the reader is referred to Ramon (1996). Another example can be found in Naples, where a 'women only' service is provided within the public sector. In the UK, there are pockets of good practice in provision of gender-sensitive services; however, most of these are provided within the voluntary or private sector. Within public sector provision in the UK, mixed wards are the norm and as a recent study showed (Johnson *et al.*, 1997), women users of mental health services are in great danger of sexual abuse and assault while in hospital. In the UK the Royal College of Nursing has campaigned for separation of the sexes in mental health facilities and also for users to have the opportunity of using the services of a nurse of the same gender.

Another dimension which is worth noting, but which has not received specific attention in this chapter, is that of ethnicity and the particular problems faced by people from ethnic minorities who use mental health services. Across Europe there have been major changes in the racial and ethnic mix with migrations from Africa and the Indian sub-continent into many countries. It is worth noting therefore that steps to make services more sensitive to gender issues should also be accompanied by moves to consider the ethnic diversity which now maintains across all European societies. As highlighted in the opening chapters, this obviously brings with it a diversity of spiritual and philosophical views which in turn have major implications for ethical frameworks.

Treatment against the patient's wishes

A recent report on London's mental health services showed that up to 50 per cent of in-patients may be detained under the Mental Health Act (Johnson *et al.*, 1997). In Europe as a whole, legislation varies widely and, in all countries, nurses are faced with the problem of detaining and treating some patients against their will. By definition these patients are in hospital when they do not want to be there and this may be for a period of assessment. However, in a majority of cases patients will be receiving some form of treatment. This treatment may involve medication or, in some cases, electroconvulsive therapy. The framework suggested by Tingle and Cribb (1995) for organizing ethical thinking and discussion is helpful in considering some of the issues. This framework contains four commonly defined key principles:

- Autonomy (the principle of respect for person's and others' right to self-determination)
- Non-maleficence (the principle not to do harm)
- Beneficence (the duty to do good)
- Justice (the principle to consider fairly the interests of all those affected) (Beauchamp and Childress, 1994).

With detention under the United Kingdom's Mental Health Act, all four of these principles need to be considered, both separately and in various combinations. The Mental Health Act 1983 has been framed in such a way that patients' rights are protected as much as possible, and there are considerable safeguards attached to the working of the Act which prevent abuses of power. Patients' rights include access to both an independent review and an appeals procedure. However, nurses, more than any other professional group, have to face the brutal reality of detaining someone in hospital who does not wish to be there. In turn, this may involve using physical restraint to prevent him or her leaving and administering injections of tranquillizing drugs against the patient's will.

Although the power of detention under the Mental Health Act lies mainly with doctors and social workers, nurses have, under Section 5 (4) of the Act, the power to detain a patient who is already receiving treatment for a mental disorder while a doctor who will consider formal detention is found. The Act makes it clear that the nurse can exercise this prerogative if he or she considers that such detention is necessary for the health or safety of the patient or for the protection of others. In addition to this formal holding power, nurses may, in many circumstances, have an important role as their view of the patient obviously influences the decision of the responsible medical officer to continue detention of a patient, to allow them to become informal, or to place another order on them. Deliberations as to whether patients are competent to make decisions about their treatment are compounded by the fact that challenges to patients' competence are often provoked when patients disagree with professionals about what is in their best interests. Nurses need to be very careful, therefore, that decisions about patient competence are kept separate from judgements about whether or not to override their decisions. In other words, would the person's competence be challenged if he or she concurred with the professional's opinion? Thus, nurses always need to ensure that the information which they provide to those responsible for making a decision is thorough, detailed and objective.

Sometimes, this will mean that although the nurse may have built a sound, trusting relationship with the patient, he or she will need to pass across information which was received in the course of that professional relationship, if it is at all relevant to the decision-making. To take one example, the patient may have confided information regarding doing harm to another person and the nurse therefore becomes duty bound to divulge that information. Thus, it may be that the principles of autonomy and non-maleficence are somewhat in conflict.

There may be occasions when nurses feel that decisions to give medication or a treatment such as ECT is wrong. Nurses should, of course, assert their view at the appropriate time, for example within a ward round or a multidisciplinary team meeting. However, in the UK, nurses have no right to conscientiously object and withdraw their services in such circumstances. Under the UKCC guidelines, nurses are obliged to take part in the treatment process.

User groups and patient autonomy

The way that nurses view autonomy has been changed considerably by the user movement within mental health services. In the United Kingdom, the user movement has grown rapidly over the last 10 years to such an extent that the last review of mental health nursing (Department of Health, 1994) published its final report under the title *Working in Partnership*, alluding to the substantial role that users of mental health services played in the review process itself. For a description of user issues specifically connected with mental health nursing, the reader is referred to Campbell (1996). Several European countries have well-developed user movements. For example, in the Netherlands there are two national organizations, the National Foundation of Patients and Residents Council and the Client Union (Baudin, 1993). These organizations have developed to become powerful in changing the attitudes of the public and professionals with regard to the rights of patients within the mental health system. The movement has certainly given the patients much greater opportunity to say what they feel about the services they are receiving and in turn, this seems to have produced positive changes in the attitudes of the professionals caring for them. Listening to patients' accounts of how they feel both about the illness they suffer and the treatment they receive is now much more central to the assessment process carried out by nurses and their fellow professionals. Indeed, the focus on personal experience has led to many services offering a much more sensitive and psychologically orientated approach to the symptoms of major mental illnesses such as schizophrenia. A Dutch psychiatrist, Marius Romme, from the University of Limburg, collected a large amount of anecdotal information from patients and together with a journalist colleague, Sandra Escher, developed a number of strategies for helping patients cope with auditory hallucinations. This work has led to the development of networks in various European countries for people who experience hallucinations and has certainly influenced the way that mental health professionals approach people with schizophrenia.

In Italy, the user movement is particularly strong and, like other European countries, has developed in parallel with relatives' organizations. Across Europe these relatives' organizations have advocated greater recognition of the carer's role and called for more information and collaboration from professionals.

The growth of the user movement and relatives' organizations across Europe has certainly led to considerable changes in the attitudes and approaches of mental health professionals. Ramon (1996) has noted that there are now user organizations in 13 European countries and the user voice is also being heard in countries of the former Eastern bloc. Prior to this recent recognition of the user perspective, patients were frequently viewed as passive recipients of the treatment process. When treatment decisions were made, the broad ethical position was of the professional adopting a paternalistic stance, making virtually all decisions on behalf of the patient and thereby largely disregarding any autonomy. The user movement has forced mental health professionals to think about the issue of treatment choice and has made them realize that decisions need to be taken from multiple perspectives, including professional knowledge, the user viewpoint, the opinions of relatives and carers and finally, the prevailing view of society. In Italy and the United Kingdom there are sizeable groups, both within and outside professional organizations, who consider that the process of deinstitutionalization has gone too far and that some patients, currently cared for in the community, should be in residential settings. This is, of course, not the only view, but it serves to emphasize that when considering overall the principle of justice within the wider societal context, professionals need to be aware that there are no simple ways of describing this dimension.

Continuing professional development

In order to provide the most effective care and treatment, continuing professional development is essential. This professional development not only includes continuing education and training but also, where at all possible, accessing skilled clinical supervision. In a sense, much continuing professional development is only made possible by the employer arranging for appropriate study leave and for access to relevant courses. Nevertheless, there is an ethical obligation on nursing staff to keep themselves abreast of developments. Nurses, as members of a profession, are responsible for updating knowledge by reading professional literature and fulfilling the duty to actively seek opportunities for enriching professional skills and knowledge. In some areas of mental health nursing this issue is more complex. For example, nurses who have received specific education and training for advanced specialist roles have a great deal of autonomy. A nurse therapist, for instance, may be referred a patient with a serious mental health problem and the referring agent will assume that the nurse applies the highest possible level of skills and knowledge.

In carrying out any psychological treatment, the individual nurse is obliged to consider issues of treatment effectiveness and, taking into account the individual assessment of the patient, must ensure that the patient is provided with the most effective treatment available. If the nurse does not have the requisite skills, there is then an obligation to ensure that treatment is available to the patient, if necessary, by another practitioner. For example, a patient may be referred to a nurse therapist for treatment of a phobic disorder which is usually treated by exposure therapy which reviews of evidence suggest is the optimum choice (Craske *et al.*, 1991). On assessment, however, it may become clear to the nurse therapist that the patient is suffering a severe level of depression and, in such a case, the evidence indicates that medication is the optimum approach. The nurse then has a clear duty either to send the patient back to the referring agent or refer him/her to an appropriately qualified person who may make a further assessment and prescribe the appropriate treatment. Clearly, while such situations are common, individual cases may pose difficulties.

An additional and obvious safeguard for nurses working in such a speciality is that of clinical supervision, which is rapidly becoming a universal standard in many European countries. Nurses have an obligation to ensure that they avail themselves of all the necessary supervisory facilities to enable them to discharge their duties in the most effective and ethical fashion and therefore supervision is demanded by the UK Council of Psychotherapy as a prerequisite to registration. In some cases, appropriate supervision may not be in place and in such circumstances nurses should act in the patient's best interests and ultimately their own best interests, by refusing to continue with the delivery of a clinical service until such facilities are made available to them. In addition, resolution of ethical problems can be greatly enhanced through the process of clinical supervision.

Elderly people

In some ways it is a pity that the topic of elderly people needs separate consideration. If society was fair, elderly people would have the same access to services and be treated in the same way as others. The reality is that in many respects, ageism is prevalent in most Western societies. In Chapter 10 Reed explores some of the reasons for ageism which are many and complex. In simple terms, older people are often perceived as less worthy of attention because of the view that their life is over and they are seen as not contributing to society, particularly in the economic sense. In addition, the cognitive decline which often accompanies old age reinforces a pre-existing negative view. Nurses are as susceptible to these negative stereotypes as are members of the general public and the detrimental effects of this are demonstrated by Norberg in her discussion of nurses working with demented patients (Chapter 3).

Nurses are often employed in positions where they have influence over equity of access and their first ethical duty is to ensure that older people are treated with the same consideration as others and that they enjoy the same access to services. There are many older people who have functional illnesses such as anxiety and depression and for whom treatments are available. The various psychotherapies and medications are as applicable and effective in older people as they are in younger age groups. Age, *per se*, should therefore never be a bar to the receipt of such treatment.

Some problems with older people, for example dementia, may lead nurses to consider both the principles of beneficence and autonomy. In the spirit of beneficence care and treatment need to be designed with an overriding concern for the ultimate benefit of the individual and, as far as possible, pay due regard to the person's power of self-determination. Nevertheless, in conditions where the patient's cognitive function is compromised, nurses may have to make paternalistic decisions on the patient's behalf. In situations where patients cannot, because of incompetence, exercise their autonomy, informed consent cannot be given. This does not mean, however, that the process of achieving consent should not be undertaken, nor does it mean that patients should not be given any information at all. Autonomy is not an absolute concept and even when it is severely restricted, there may well be certain areas of daily life about which patients are able to make decisions.

The cognitive impairment which may be present in many cases will affect how much information is given to the patient and in which mode. Those caring for older people should always err on the side of caution and respect for personhood and, therefore, it is always better to give the patient too much information rather than too little, even though some of it may be beyond their comprehension. Unfortunately, there is widespread evidence that some of those involved in the care of older people err on the wrong side and provide little or no information, assuming that the cognitive impairment is such that the person will not be able to understand anything. Once more, nursing practice should be guided by both the multi-disciplinary team and the process of supervision.

With regard to older people with dementing illnesses who are being cared for in hospital, the same principles apply as to those patients who are detained under the Mental Health Act for treatment of a serious and enduring illness such as schizophrenia. There are many occasions when the nurse may well have to take action which is contrary to the patient's wishes to ensure that either they, or others, are not harmed. To take a common example, the nurse may need to physically restrain a patient from leaving hospital to protect him or her from being knocked over on a busy road.

Returning to an earlier point, the care of older people should, in the vast majority of respects, be subject to the same ethical principles as that for any other age group.

Conclusion

Mental health nursing is a profession which embraces a wide range of skills, roles and responsibilities. The ethical challenges posed for practitioners in caring for some of society's most vulnerable people are therefore many and varied. New roles in the community, such as those of case managers, are producing new dilemmas, particularly in the area of public safety. It seems likely that mental health legislation will change across Europe, as the provision of compulsory treatment in the community becomes increasingly necessary.

Furthermore, it is likely that nurses will have new powers of detention and treatment at their disposal. The ethical problems which come with these new responsibilities will be great. On account of this, there is a need to strengthen multidisci-plinary teamwork, so that nurses may experience and benefit from the necessary support. Recent work (Onyett *et al.*, 1995) suggests that community mental health teams still, by and large, function at a suboptimal level and there may be real problems in achieving best nursing practice. These problems are by no means confined to the United Kingdom as community teams are a relatively new development world-wide. An additional safeguard for nurses is access to skilled supervision, where ethical problems may be shared and a solution found.

Having said all that, one needs to consider the wide variation in standards of mental health nursing across Europe. Following the 'Velvet Revolution' in the former Czechoslovakia, I undertook a trip to take part in a training exercise held in Prague and in the countryside of what is now the Czech Republic. I was truly taken aback by the way that the mental health services in that country appeared to be out of date, even when compared with the standards which maintained at the beginning of my training in the late 1960s. However, on returning to that country on several occasions in the ensuing five years, the training and the attitude of the workforce have changed beyond all recognition.

The Czech Republic now has a workforce of psychiatrists, psychologists and nurses who are developing innovations in community care and who have made up many of the deficits in education and attitude attributable to the four decades of communist repression. The situation in other former Eastern European countries, however, is still very mixed. While user organizations flourish in Hungary and Poland, countries such as Romania still care for the mentally ill in sometimes squalid and medieval conditions. Although there are many examples of doctors and nurses who are attempting to bring Romania's mental health services to a reasonable level, the nursing workforce is largely ignorant of modern pharmacological or psychotherapeutic approaches.

In situations such as these, some of the more sophisticated ethical considerations referred to above have little or no relevance. Many patients are not receiving the most basic level of care and there are few, if any, resources for education and training. There is currently one training initiative led by a team from the Maudsley Hospital and the Institute of Psychiatry which includes notable figures from British mental health such as Ray Rowden, Victoria Hornby and Jim Birley, but such initiatives need to be replicated. There is, in the author's view, a responsibility for those of us in richer developed countries to do more than offer wise words. Countries such as Romania do not only need financial aid, but also education and training from more fortunate workforces. Perhaps the final message of this chapter should be that the responsibility for providing ethically sound mental health services across the world is a responsibility that we should all share.

References

Battaglia, G. (1987) 'The expanding role of the nurse and the contracting role of the hospital in Italy', *International Journal of Social Psychiatry*, **33**: 115–18.

Baudin, D. (1993) *A Guide To Mental Health Care*. (Survivors Speak Out: London).

Beauchamp, T.L. and Childress, J.F. (1994) *Principles of Biomedical Ethics*, 4th edn. (Oxford University Press: New York).

British Psychological Society (1995) *Professional Practice Guidelines*. (Division of Clinical Psychology of the British Psychological Society: Leicester).

Campbell, P. (1996) 'Working with service users', in Sandford, T. and Gournay, K. (eds) *Perspectives in Mental Health Nursing*. (Baillière Tindall: London), pp. 5–16.

Craske, M., Rapee, R. and Barlow, D. (1991) 'Cognitive behavioural treatment of panic disorder, agoraphobia and generalised anxiety disorder', in Turner, S., Calhoun, K. and Adams, H. (eds) *Handbook of Clinical Behaviour Therapy*, 2nd edn. (John Wiley: New York), pp. 39–66.

Decker, J., Goris, C. and Sanders, H. (1995) *Zergcoordinatie en Revalidatie in de Psychiatrie*, Onderzoek and Ontwikkeling and Opleiding. (Publikataties Psychiatrish Ziekenhuis: Amsterdam).

Department of Health (1989) *Caring for People with Mental Illness: The Care Programme Approach*. (HMSO: London).

Department of Health (1991) *Working together under the Children Act 1989: a guide to arrangements for interagency cooperation for the protection of children from abuse*. (HMSO: London).

Department of Health (1994) *Working in Partnership – A Review of Mental Health Nursing*. (HMSO: London).

Department of Health (1995) *The Report of the Clinical Standards Advisory Group on Schizophrenia*. (HMSO: London).

Filson, P. and Kendrick, T. (1997) 'Survey of roles of CPNs and occupational therapists', *Psychiatric Bulletin*, **21**(2): 70–3.

Gournay, K.J.M. (1996) *No Panic: A Practical Guide to Managing Panic and Phobia*. (Asset Books: Surrey).

Johnson S., Ramsay, R. and Thornicroft, G. (1997) *London's Mental Health: A Report to the King's Fund London Commission*. (King's Fund: London).

Lancashire, S., Haddock, G., Tarrier, N. *et al.* (1997) 'Effects of training in psychosocial interventions for CPNs in England', *Psychiatric Services*, **48**(1): 39–41.

Marks, I. (1985) *Nurse Therapists in Primary Care.* (RCN: London).

Marks, I., Connelly, J., Hallam, R. and Philpott, R. (1977) *Nursing in Behavioural Psychotherapy.* (RCN: London).

Moore, S. (1961) 'A psychiatric outpatient nursing service', *Mental Health Bulletin*, **20**: 51–4.

Mosher, L. and Burti, L. (1994) *Community Mental Health.* (Norton: New York).

O'Halloran, P., Gournay, K. and Whiting, D. (1995) 'Clinical case management. Training practice and implementation issues: an Australian example', in Decker, J., Goris, C. and Sanders, H., *Zorgcoordinatie en Revalidatie in de Psychiatrie*, Onderzoek and Ontwikkeling and Opleiding (Publikataties Psychiatrish Ziekenhuis: Amsterdam).

Onyett, S., Pillinger, T. and Muijen, M. (1995) *Making Community Mental Health Teams Work.* (Sainsbury Centre Publications: London).

Pfeiffer, J. (1993) 'Mental health reforms in the Czech Republic', in Dean, C. and Freeman, H. (eds) *Community Mental Health Care.* (Gaskell: London).

Ramon, S. (1996) *Mental Health in Europe.* (Mind Publications: London).

Ritchie, J., Dick, D. and Lingham, R. (1994) *Report of the Enquiry into the Care and Treatment of Christopher Clunis.* (HMSO: London).

Sainsbury Centre for Mental Health (1997) *Pulling Together: The Future Roles and Training of Mental Health Staff.* (Sainsbury Centre Publications: London).

Tingle, J. and Cribb, A. (1995) *Nursing Law and Ethics.* (Blackwell Science: Oxford).

United Kingdom Central Council for Nursing, Midwifery and Health Visiting (UKCC) (1992) *Code of Professional Conduct for Nurses, Midwives and Health Visitors.* (UKCC: London).

Suggestions for further reading

Barker, P. and Baldwin, S. (1991) *Ethical Issues in Mental Health.* (Chapman & Hall: London).

British Psychological Society Division of Clinical Psychology (1995) *Professional Practice Guidelines.* (BPS Publications: Leicester).

Fairburn, G.J. (1995) *Contemplating Suicide: The Language of Ethics and Self Harm.* (Routledge: London).

Perkins, R. and Repper, J. (1996) *Working alongside People with Long Term Mental Health Problems.* (Chapman & Hall: London).

Ramon, S. (1985) *Psychiatry in Britain.* (Croom Helm: Beckenham).

10

Ethical Issues in the Care of Older People: Difference, Distinction and Division

Jan Reed

Introduction

Ethical debates about the care of older people are extremely interesting on a range of dimensions. They evoke ideas about justice, fairness, personhood and rights, among other things, but one of the fundamental issues which is not often made explicit is the degree to which the concerns that we raise are actually about ourselves. With some of the client groups identified in this book, we can see or construct some clear divisions between these groups and others and between these groups and ourselves. When we talk about children, for example, we can use some legally determined or empirically researched chronological age as a cut-off point. Below this, humans are children and above this, they are not. When talking about people with mental health problems we can use some diagnostic classification system or assessment schedule to say whether or not a person belongs to a particular group. There are, however, problems with these lines of demarcation: individual variations in development make childhood a more elastic concept than we suppose and mental health problems have to be placed in an ever-changing context of cultural definitions and norms. Nevertheless, these definitions are used and part of their function is not only to specify the characteristics, needs and problems of particular client groups, but also to distinguish them from 'us', the professionals, the normal people.

In the case of older people this will not do. While it is possible to point to legal definitions of, say, 'pensionable age', empirical evidence does not support the idea that there are clear developmental changes once this age is reached. Individual variations and differences are too marked to make this credible. Not only is it difficult, therefore, to demarcate older people, separate them from other client groups and specify their unique needs and problems, but it also becomes difficult to separate them from ourselves. Older people are us, just a bit further on in development and experience. We will become old, we will become them. Being old is not like being young, something you grow out of, it is what everyone will grow into. Being old is not a time-limited condition, like being pregnant, nor is it something for which there might be a cure, like mental illness, it is just being old. When we debate ethical issues in the care of older people, therefore, we debate our own care.

Historically, for professionals such as nurses, the demarcation lines between patient and professional have been an important part of our role and social identity. Menzies (1960) described how much nursing work at the time of her study was based around routines which served to depersonalize care and create a distance between nurse and patient. Armstrong (1983), in his analysis of the nurse–patient relationship, describes how, until the 1970s, many nursing textbooks concentrated almost exclusively on the technical and manual aspects of nursing. When 'psychology' was mentioned, the nurse–patient relationship was often portrayed not as something which was in any way intimate, but instead centred on the nurse as a model of health and efficiency who would inspire patients to comply with their treatment regimes. To some extent, things have changed with the development of more personalized approaches to care, such as the nursing process, patient-centred nursing models and ideas of holistic care. At an official level, at least, nurses appear to be moving towards a more personalized form of care in which emotional closeness is more valued than it was and has ceased to be something to be strenuously avoided.

Distance has also been maintained by language, in the way that this has emphasized difference and has also become pejorative. It is easy to dismiss issues of language as trivial, when in fact they are extremely important because language not only reflects, but also shapes, what we feel (Reed and Ground, 1996). Referring to older people as 'geriatrics', for example, reduces them to examples of a medical speciality, while the term 'the elderly' emphasizes their distinctness as a group. Looking back over the years at my own work, I shudder with embarrassment about the words that I have used. The use of the fairly recent term 'older people', makes the point that there is a group which simply consists of people who are older than others. Critics point out that everyone is older than someone else but in some ways, this is a positive aspect of the term. For instance, it reminds me that I am older than some people, that you are older than some people and that we all share this state of seniority. Most importantly, there is some evidence that older people themselves prefer this term (Walker, 1993).

These issues of difference and distinction are the central themes of this chapter. If ethics is about anything, it is about how we treat each other and how others treat us; put simply, it is about shared experiences and values. Making distinctions and differences is therefore at the heart of ethical debate – do our distinctions allow the needs and problems of our fellow human beings to be addressed more effectively, or do they simply create unhelpful divisions which are ultimately unethical in themselves?

Opinion is very much divided on this. At a pragmatic level, it seems obvious that meeting needs depends on being able to identify them and this is facilitated by being able to classify and summarize the groups of people who have these needs. This process also raises a number of concerns. Many writers have made the point that some policies based on differentiating older people from others result in them being separated from others in physical and social ways, such as receiving care in, for example, care homes or hospitals, or by being excluded from social activities and debates. Retirement policies and pensions for older people are an interesting example of this process. Pensions which are provided simply on the basis of a person reaching a particular age seem to be benevolent mechanisms for ensuring provision for older people. When they are interpreted by employers as a rationale for compulsory retirement their benevolence becomes questionable as they are then being used as an excuse to exclude older people from the job market. Because pensions are not equal to salaries, older people inevitably experience reduced incomes which affect their activities and participation in social events. Older people become 'hidden' from others, they are not seen around and, therefore, their experiences are not acknowledged in everyday discussions. Another way of hiding the structured inequalities experienced by older people is by portraying them as affluent and emphasizing the power of the 'grey pound'. As Ginn (1993) points out, this process denies the problems that older people face.

Often, these issues can be seen most easily at the political and policy levels where issues of distinction materialize into legislation, funding decisions and service provision (Hugman, 1996). When comparing different countries, as in this book, there are obvious advantages in concentrating on this level of debate as policies are more available to scrutiny than individual personal debates. Also, information about professional concerns can be very limited, particularly if, as in the case of the care of older people, the nursing input is not always significant and the professional voice is not always heard. This does not mean, however, that the ethical issues covered in this chapter will only be at a political or policy level. What I hope to explore is the relationship between this form of ethical debate and the delivery of care. Nursing takes place in political and social contexts which shape practice in powerful ways and an awareness of this dynamic is essential if nursing is to understand and develop practice. To see nursing ethics as distinct from the general political and social context in which nurses work, is to miss an opportunity to identify and voice concerns, to challenge prevailing assumptions and to ensure that the care that we give is consistent with our professional values and those of our clients.

Ethical issues at a policy level

The areas of moral and political philosophy are important in this discussion. These areas have often been considered as distinct from each other in general textbooks of philosophy where, for example, there are separate chapters for each topic. In philosophical writings this distinction is not always clear, however, and philosophers such as Kant or Mill discuss general principles of conduct which they apply to both personal and political spheres. It is useful, however, to make some distinction between the two topics, based on the recognition that there is a great deal of difference between the state and an individual (Reed and Ground, 1996). There is, of course, a relationship between the two – the state acts for or represents individuals, ignores them or oppresses them. Equally, individuals have varying degrees of influence on state activities.

The decisions that are made at a political level, therefore, impact on practice and care. This may be in the way that resources and funding for care are determined, the way that priorities for spending are set, or the way in which goals and aims for services are formulated (Boyajian, 1988). Where state resources are limited, always remembering that the state has already made decisions about what level of resources it should have, through its taxation policies, then the competing claims of various different groups have to be weighed against each other. In this process of weighing, a number of considerations are possible. First, it may be thought that the state does not have a responsibility to meet these needs, that the provision of state support is either demeaning to people because it reduces their independence, or it is unjust to those who have been prudent enough to make their own provision. Second, if some state responsibility is acknowledged, then a number of other considerations come into play about the strength of the claims of different groups.

Cultural and social values influence how decisions between the claims of different groups are made. Societies can, for example, attach merit to certain groups because their dependency arises from an activity which is approved of. War heroes are usually regarded more highly than drug addicts because the former group acquired their disability through activities which were of benefit to others in society, while the latter group can be reviled because their problems are seen as self-inflicted and of no benefit to others and indeed may make others' lives more uncomfortable, unpleasant or dangerous. Decision-making of this type evokes notions of reciprocity, that is, the idea that the contributions that a group of people make (or have made in the past) should be rewarded and met with equivalent contributions. If this form of reciprocity prevails, older people are likely to benefit as their past military, political and cultural contributions – in a Europe which, in this century, has seen much conflict – will be held up as justification for providing them with support now. If, however, the idea of reciprocity is time limited, so that only current contributions are acknowledged, then the position of older people becomes more vulnerable. If older people are not working or fulfilling active social or familial roles, then they can be seen as parasites on the active, working, money-making, younger population.

Another temporal dimension of reciprocity is the commitment that we might feel to future generations. As Becker (1986) has argued, this is a somewhat puzzling idea which seems to be based on some sort of allegiance to the notion that perpetuating the human race (or at least our own ethnic version of it) is of great importance. Another element of this commitment to future generations is perhaps based on self-interest, in that we look after the young so that they will look after us if we need help when we are old. It may be the case that, when choosing between meeting the needs of older people or those of children and younger people, one conception of reciprocity would lead us to favour future generations. The irony is, of course, that if this is done for reasons of self-interest then we abandon older people in the hope that younger people will not do the same to us in the future.

There are, of course, other cultural values which impinge upon the decisions made about the distribution of resources to different groups. For example, Western society is often described as being youth-orientated, in the way that people see youth as desirable and old age as distasteful. This set of values can make older people an unpopular choice for resource allocation. These negative attitudes to others have been explored by many writers who point to reflections of these aesthetics in both literature and current cultural images (Till, 1993; Blaikie, 1994). As Norman (1987) has put it, 'both as individuals and as members of society, we find it extremely difficult to be honest about our attitudes to old age and old people. There is an ambivalence at the root of our being.' Norman details this ambivalence further when she talks about feelings which 'cannot with decency be openly expressed' such as '[the] contempt of the young and strong for the old and weak; fear of the mortality which old age represents; guilt which is translated into anger; and resentment over the need to use scarce resources and precious time on people "who have had their life"' (Norman, 1987, p. 3).

The 'unpopularity' of older people in Europe very much depends on them being singled out as a group of people who are different from the rest of us. This demarcation simultaneously creates and reinforces stereotypes of older people and puts in place mechanisms for systematically classifying their needs as being the problems of old age, rather than problems which are shared across society. What seems a reasonable and sensible approach to identifying need can become a means of pigeonholing people and reducing them to stereotypes. Whether we adopt a position of 'compassionate ageism' (Binstock, 1984) where we feel pity for the frailty and problems of older people, or whether we portray them more positively as affluent and therefore less needy, approaching what Arber and Ginn (1991) have termed 'conflictual ageism', where older people are seen as taking resources away from other groups, both of these positions depend on stereotypes.

It was these concerns that prompted the 1993 'European Year of Older People and Solidarity between Generations'. The aims of the year were, by and large, to highlight the ways in which older people in Europe were living their lives and, perhaps more importantly, to foster mutual understanding across generations and identify areas of common or mutual concern, rather than differences.

Ethical issues at a practice level

The above discussion about wide-ranging social and political ethical debates might appear to be about issues which are separate from nursing care. These issues do, however, impinge upon nursing practice in a number of ways. The ethical and political framework of resource allocation and policy development provides the context in which practice takes place.

Perhaps the most obvious way in which this happens is in the way that the value accorded to particular client groups affects the resources that nurses can command. The label 'Cinderella service' is evidence of this and is frequently applied to such client groups as older people and people who have learning difficulties or mental health problems. These resources affect the material state of the buildings in which care is delivered, whether there are carpets on the floor, the quality of the curtains and the equipment available. Resources also determine the number of staff that are available, the degree to which they are trained and, to some extent, the amount that they are paid. Seedhouse (1988) touches on this in his 'ethical grid' through which he develops a framework for making ethical decisions. He includes in one layer of the grid (the black layer in his diagram) a range of external considerations about the law, codes of practice and the wishes of others, which all impinge on ethical decision-making. As Seedhouse argues, 'in many cases, in the real hard world, the black layer contains the most important factors of all' (Seedhouse, 1988, p. 138).

More subtly, political decisions about the importance and value of older people affect the goals and aims of nursing care. Evers (1981) has evocatively described an ethos of care which she called 'warehousing', where older people were 'stored' in geriatric wards until they died. Evers points out the lack of therapy and rehabilitation in these environments and the pervasive view that the function of the care service was to do little more than this. This state of affairs owes much to the negative and pessimistic views of older people which seem almost endemic in many cultures, the way that they are translated into policies which set organizational goals and into the practices which operationalize these goals. While many nursing debates tend to be carried out as if they were separate from the prevailing political and organizational contexts, a number of studies suggest that there is a close relationship between organizational goals and values and the nursing care given to older people (Baker, 1983; Reed, 1989).

Looking at some of the values and goals of nursing, it is evident not only that organizational goals can shape practice, but also where this impetus does not correspond with nursing ethics, then conflicts can arise. Take, for example, the nursing goal of individualized care with its connotations of respect for persons. This can be operationalized through a range of different nursing activities, such as acting as an advocate for older people. As Kendrick (1997) points out, however, acting as an advocate is an idea with inherent problems surrounding issues of power. Moreover, in an organization or health care system which is not supportive of the wishes of patients, does not respect their autonomy and is simply trying to deliver care as cheaply as possible, the role of advocate is ultimately unsuccessful and may raise expectations only to see them dashed.

Linking policy and practice debates

Macintyre's (1977) analysis of policy for older people provides a useful framework in which to examine these connections more closely. She points out that the idea of old age as a social problem which needs to be addressed through policy and provision is a relatively recent phenomenon in the UK. Throughout early policy developments for dealing with the needy such as the Elizabethan Poor Laws, older people were not distinguished in any way from other groups of people needing support or 'relief'. Macintyre argues that they only became 'officially' recognized in policy formation towards the end of the nineteenth century and there is some evidence (see Troyansky, 1996 for an overview) that this was the case in other European countries.

When older people were distinguished as a special group of the poor and needy, Macintyre argues that this was tied up with ideas about 'deserving and undeserving' poor. Some of the strategies for dealing with need, such as 'indoor' or workhouse relief, were partly designed and administered as ways of discouraging people from applying for help and as a means of motivating them to provide for themselves. As such, the strategy was based on the assumption that many of the poor were able to fend for themselves, but were too lazy or dissolute to do so (Longmate, 1974). Older people, however, could not be accused of such moral degeneracy as even the most vigorous detective of abuses of the public purse could see that older people were simply not capable of providing for themselves, particularly in a world where the Industrial

Revolution had put a heavy premium on hard manual labour in factories.

Macintyre further discusses how, after the identification of older people as a social problem, the problem itself is open to different formulations. The first formulation is that the problem is a humanitarian one, in other words 'a perception of old age as bringing problems of various kinds to individuals, problems which the community should attempt to ameliorate through increased provision' (Macintyre, 1977, p. 49). She goes on to argue that the humanitarian view was the one which predominated in the UK at the beginning of this century. It stimulated the separation of older people from other needy groups and set policy goals as being the appropriate and adequate provision of support.

Macintyre then goes on to describe how the problem of old age was reformulated as the century progressed. This was particularly evident as the debates in the UK about the new Welfare State took place and plans for this were developed. Beveridge, for example, more than once cautioned against too-liberal provision for older people as the Welfare State that he envisaged would be funded through the contributions of young working people, and therefore their welfare was paramount. The problem of old age became one of how to reduce their demands on others, or how to meet their needs at a containable (and reduced) cost. Macintyre describes this as the organizational perspective, 'consideration of how best to reduce the social costs imposed on the community by the elderly population' (p. 44).

If we use this framework as a way of exploring the impact of policy on practice, then we can look at three sets of implications. First, if the policy formulation is a humanitarian one, then the goals of care are to meet need and address problems in as effective a way as possible. The concern is primarily that older people are not receiving enough care, or care of an adequate standard. The expectations of such a formulation, therefore, would be that resources would be made available, or at least efforts would be made to provide them. There would also be concerns about the quality of the care that was delivered and that it was provided in the right way and at the right time. Because this would, hopefully, entail some concern for the views of older people themselves, then it is also reasonable to expect that the autonomy of older people would be promoted, as would the nurses' role as advocate.

If, however, the policy formulation is an organizational one and the central concern is to minimize cost, then practice is very different. Not only are the resources for care limited, but the whole goal of the service is to provide minimum standards of care within these minimum resources. Practice becomes a matter of scrimping and saving, with few staff and little equipment. To use Evers' phrase, the goals of care are about 'warehousing'. Ethical practice, which might include the promotion of autonomy and the development of advocacy roles, becomes extremely difficult to establish and nurses who adopt these values find them difficult to put into practice.

We must not forget, however, the other state of affairs that Macintyre describes which is the state where old age is not identified as a social problem at all. While the humanitarian formulation can be seen as a positive approach and the organizational one can be regarded as a negative approach, both depend on making a distinction between older people and everyone else. If we accept the argument that such distinctions inevitably create barriers between people and foster stereotypical thinking, then we are coming close to arguing that they are inherently unethical in a way that erodes respect for persons as unique individuals, reducing them to stark demographic characteristics. If this line of reasoning is followed, the conclusion that making distinctions is inherently a bad thing if we want to practise ethically, must be drawn.

Alternatively, not making distinctions may lead to other ethical problems. Treating older people just like everyone else fails to delineate the particular issues that face them and that may require specific action. In that case, one must conclude that not making distinctions is inherently a bad thing if we want to practise ethically.

Ethical issues in the care of older people: a European perspective

So far, this chapter has tried to explore ideas about the ways in which political and policy decisions are ultimately based on judgements of value and therefore are inescapably linked to ethical debates. In particular, there has been some debate on the ethical consequences of distinguishing between older people and everyone else. This distinction can be the basis of prob-lematizing older people in ways that can be broadly regarded as either positive, or negative, in their consequences. These consequences arise from the way that solutions are posed and by the impact that these solutions have on practice.

From this we can begin to postulate some ethical dilemmas and issues for nurses and we can now extend the discussion to an examination of the issues from a European perspective. In the introduction to this chapter I suggested that one way to explore ethical issues in the care of older people in other countries was to look at the policies that they have. This is because policies are often more accessible than professional debates, especially where professional input into the care of older people may be minimal or difficult to identify. Using Macintyre's useful framework, I now want to concentrate on the idea of distinguishing between older people and the rest of society as a fundamental ethical debate. To do so, it is neces-sary to identify, as far as possible, countries where this distinc-tion is not made. Under these circumstances it is impossible to identify professional debates as there can be no professional debate specifically about the care of older people if older people are not identified as a specific group of people needing care.

The following discussion, while it draws where possible on material which is directly about the ethical debates facing nurses caring for older people across Europe, also makes significant use of the available information about general policies and polit-ical philosophies in these countries. The connection between practice and policy, therefore, is made as much by deduction and postulation as by empirical evidence.

Denmark: the humanitarian formulation

Denmark is, perhaps, one of the European countries that comes closest to a strong humanitarian formulation of the 'problem' of old age. The chief concerns of provision and practice seem to be to provide the best possible care for older people. Johansen

(1986) charts the history of welfare provision in Denmark which in many ways is similar to the UK history. A series of Poor Laws and workhouse systems did not distinguish between older people and other needy groups until the end of the nineteenth century when the Old Age Relief Act was enacted in 1891 (Johansen, 1986). Early in the twentieth century, however, a series of reforms, such as the 1922 Old Age Pension Reform and the 1933 Social Reform, which introduced universal benefits, established welfare provision for older people in advance of UK developments.

Denmark has also been quicker than the UK to move towards community care and the provision of care for older people in their own homes. Indeed, Jamieson (1990) notes that there is no equivalent term for 'community care' in the Danish language, which she suggests indicates a lack of ambiguity about the nature of care. It is assumed that it will be community based and hence needs no further qualification. While standards of care in institutional settings are high, no additional care homes have been built since the Housing for the Elderly Act of 1987 and the emphasis has been on providing care to older people in their own homes. To this end, the building of specialized accommodation has been encouraged as have a wide range of facilities and home-based services, including gardening and snow-clearing (Wilderom, 1991). This move, which Giarchi describes as in some ways resembling the 'brave Italian decision to close down its psychiatric institutions' (Giarchi, 1996, p. 99), seems to have been prompted less by overt concerns about the cost of provision than by the desire to respect the wishes and preferences of older people (Abrahamson, 1991). Nevertheless, as predictions for population growth suggest that by the year 2025 the proportion of older people will be 22.2 per cent, which is the second highest in Europe, issues of cost and the sustainability of provision are raised.

With this long history of well-established provision it is not surprising that suggestions for reductions in provision and/or dismantling of the Welfare State have been met with great unease (Giarchi, 1996). The welfare system in Denmark, as Jamieson (1990) describes it, is almost completely state-managed, with very little voluntary or private sector involvement. There is little desire to change this or to put more responsibility on to family networks as state provision is seen as a right of citizens and no stigma is attached to using these services (Jamieson, 1990; Giarchi, 1996).

In accordance with these beliefs and principles, the most frequently voiced criticism of the system is the degree to which it provides a high quality of service which meets the needs of older people – the humanitarian formulation of the problem of old age. Jamieson (1990), listing some of the concerns which have been voiced, identified that some people are being hospitalized needlessly and that professionals tend to exclude them from participation in decision-making. Jamieson also indicates that social aspects of care, such as social contact and integration, are also missing from Danish care, a situation which she suggests may be seen as 'inherent in the professional approach which characterises the public services' (p. 13).

For the practitioner, the ethical issues of caring for older people in Denmark are not centrally concerned with establishing and maintaining rights to care or equity of provision, at least not at the moment. The ethical concerns are, by and large, about how this care can be improved. One particular area of concern seems to be the degree to which older people are empowered and their autonomy supported and respected. Ramhoej (1992), for example, has described how in nursing home care, 'great importance is attached to attitudes towards elderly people living in homes. The old person should not lose their civic rights when moving to an old people's home. His room is his residence and should be regarded as sacred' (p. 17). The rights of citizenship, which convey entitlement to services, need to be extended to rights within the service such as rights to shape care, to have some say in how it is given and what form it should take. Ramhoej also goes on to describe how personnel should not 'undertake responsibility' for the older person but 'the person himself decides which offers [of help] he wishes' (p. 17). This may involve some form of advocacy at an individual rather than at a societal level, but nurses need to make an effort to find out what it is that older people want and then establish how and if it can be managed.

The United Kingdom – the organizational formulation

The UK situation comes closest to the organizational formulation than to any other, although none of these forms is 'pure'. Macintyre (1977) points out that there has always been some ambivalence in UK attitudes towards provision for older people, and this is evident even in policies which are generally felt to be humanitarian. Beveridge, for example, in the Report of 1942 which paved the way for the Welfare State, sums up the problem thus: 'On the one hand, the provision made for age must be satisfactory otherwise great numbers may suffer. On the other hand, every shilling added to pension rates is extremely costly in total... It is dangerous to be in any way lavish to old age, until adequate provision has been assured for all other needs, such as the prevention of disease and the adequate nutrition of the young' (Beveridge, 1942, para. 236).

This ambivalence continues to the present day, although more recently the concerns being voiced about the care of older people seem to be more clearly organizational, as the demographic time bomb is predicted to explode in the near future, showering the UK with older people who will be a drain on resources. Debates about resources often involve discussion of people's responsibility to provide for themselves through, for example, personal pension plans. Recent pension scandals where people have been misled about the returns from schemes, or where funds have been embezzled, have raised some questions about this move. Similarly, moves to encourage the participation of families in the care of older people may reduce the burden on the state, but in practical terms, many families may not be able or willing to provide this care, nor may older people be happy to accept it.

In this climate of encouraging individual responsibility, the state has not remained completely inactive, on the contrary, a wide-ranging review of health and social services for everyone has been undertaken in recent years. There has been an explicit encouragement of more voluntary and private sector involvement in provision, for example through stipulations that local authorities spend a certain proportion of their budgets purchasing services from this sector (Giarchi, 1996). This idea of creating a 'welfare mix' so that the state, the private sector, voluntary organizations and individuals combine to provide services is an attempt to move away from what is often seen as a rigid and bureaucratic state-controlled system which fails to meet clients' or consumers' needs. The other side of the coin, however, is that consumerism can only work if consumers have the power to purchase, that is, they have resources at their disposal. For those who have been unable to save money or accumulate wealth, or who have only minimum pensions, purchasing power is just a dream.

The ethical issues for nurses in the organizational formulation are mainly concerned with maintaining equity and justice in the allocation of resources. If the organizational solutions that are proposed are to move responsibility from the state to the individual, as seems to be the case in the UK proposals, then the ethical issues facing practitioners are about rights to services. Whereas one view would be that these rights should only be dependent on the ability to pay for services, this is not the only view and nurses need to explore and articulate other rationales such as respect for persons, the idea of basic human rights and the ideas of justice.

Bosnia and the former Yugoslavia – no formulation

It is difficult to imagine a society or culture in Europe which has not identified the 'problem' of old age in one way or another, or which has not at least marked out older people in some way. The ideal of a society where age does not matter in the way that people are regarded is one that may seem attractive to those who have seen or experienced the harmful effects of ageism. Reading accounts of workhouse life prior to the 'official' recognition of old age, where everyone was treated alike regardless of the reasons behind their destitution and need, does suggest that making a special case of old age may well have some benefits. To do otherwise is to revert to a horrendous form of 'jungle law' where older people are accorded no concessions in the struggle for survival. Before older people were formally recognized as different from other groups of needy people, they were required to work alongside other fitter inmates at what were sometimes arduous tasks and were given no concessions in the provision of food or accommodation (Longmate, 1974).

Trying to explore the ethical consequences of non-discrimination in contemporary European culture is a difficult task because the idea of age as a primary means of describing people is such a powerful and pervasive one. There is some evidence, however, that in some European cultures the notion of age as an important way of categorizing people is relatively weak and this raises questions about how this translates into care.

A research study carried out in Bosnia has suggested that the category of 'elderly' is not a meaningful social category. 'There is a simple absence of such a cognitive category in many Bosnian people's understanding of their society' (Vincent and Mudrovcic, 1993, p. 98). In response to the authors' questions about the problems older people had in Bosnia, the frequent reply was that they had the same problems as everyone else.

This does not mean that the life course is not conceptualized in any way in Bosnian culture, but rather that chronological age is not the foundational idea. Instead, Vincent and Mudrovcic identify the recurring idea of *snaga*, which they translate as power or vigour, so that old age involves a loss of *snaga*. When older people were asked about how they felt about ageing, their response was often that they had lost their *snaga*.

The cultural context of *snaga* is explained by Vincent and Mudrovcic in relation to established lifestyles in Bosnia, particularly in the rural areas. Work, mainly consisting of farm labour, is synonymous with life for many people. As Vincent and Mudrovcic describe it, 'work in this sense is not the British concept of paid employment but rather the activities in the house, on the land, in the factory or workshop necessary for survival' (1993, p. 99). This integration of work and life is perhaps a reflection of the stage of industrialization which Bosnia has reached. As Vincent and Mudrovcic point out, migration from rural to urban areas has only been a significant feature over the last 30 years and in rural communities the pattern of life is built on shared family households and agricultural activities. In this environment formal retirement ages mean little and the integration of generations in collaborative working means that *snaga* is more salient than age. With the movement to urban areas, such patterns, while remaining strong cultural templates, have shifted and increasingly younger people are moving to towns to new forms of work, leaving older people in rural areas. The differences between generations are therefore inextricably linked to differences in work and location.

Nevertheless, the notion of *snaga* rather than chronological age being a more important marker of life is an appealing one in many ways. The loss of strength, while it may occur mainly in older people, is not unique to them and this opens up the possibility of solidarity across generations between all those with debilitating conditions. Similarly, for those older people who do not experience a loss of *snaga*, the social stereotypes of older people may not be applied to them in a draconian and inflexible way. In this way, physical condition becomes more important than age as a social category, a situation which seems more fair, logical and helpful.

When the translation of this into policy and service provision is considered, however, some problems arise, particularly in the context of the violent upheavals in the former Yugoslavia. The communist regime, with its superficial motto of 'brotherhood and unity' espoused by the totalitarian leader Tito, collapsed with his death. This collapse and the ensuing ethnic conflict resulted in the demolition of the centralized communist policy-making machine (Giarchi, 1996). In such an environment, if the needs of specific groups are not acknowledged and their importance reinforced, they can easily be forgotten.

Giarchi (1996) argues that many older people in the former Yugoslavia are experiencing great deprivation. Pensions, for those that have access to them, are not always paid in full or on time because of war conditions. Ruzica *et al.* (1991) suggest that the poverty of older people receiving pensions is partly due to their low level in an economic climate where inflation at one point in 1989 was 1365 per cent, leading to a situation where at least half of the older people were below the poverty line. It is not surprising, then, that significant numbers of older people stay at work. In 1985 the figure was 20 per cent, with half of this group working full time, but with internal wars, opportunities for employment are likely to be very much reduced.

Services for older people are very difficult to evaluate, particularly since the wars began. Giarchi's summary of discussing nursing services and nursing homes illustrates this well when he states that 'little has been published regarding the numbers involved, eligibility and the extent and quality of the work' (1996, p. 420). In discussing mental health care, Giarchi simply states that there are 'no reports available regarding mental health services for older people in the territories of the former Yugoslavia' (p. 421). Nevertheless there is some information available which gives some indication about the level of provision. Ruzica *et al.* (1991) state that institutional care, when provided at all, is based in a small number of homes (less than 200 across the former Yugoslavia), each with between 150 and 200 residents and, at the time of publication, at least 5400 people on the waiting list.

There is some evidence that even before the wars this provision was being cut back (Giarchi, 1996) and the care of older people was being returned to the family sphere, alongside the movement towards decentralization and away from traditional state institutions (Milosavljevic and Ruzica, 1989). This reliance on family care echoes the recent rural past where families tended to work and live together with the general expectation that the family, rather than the state, should bear this responsibility. Giarchi quotes Article 124 of the Law of Marriage and Family Relations in Slovenia as an example of this: 'Children of age are obliged to maintain their parents who are incapable of work or do not have enough means for their care' (Giarchi, 1996, p. 426). While this emphasis on family values may seem right and proper to some, it must be remembered that if society as a whole does not take responsibility for older people and families break up, as in the case of war, older people are left to fend for themselves or to receive help from voluntary agencies, such as the Red Cross (Giarchi, 1996). With the extreme form of decentralization found in the break-up of the former Yugoslavia where a centralized communist regime has been replaced by a range of warring factions fighting over territory and resources, a 'rather anarchic' political scene ensues with 'enterprises... becoming increasingly exposed to open markets [and] there is no special protection by the state, close downs are more and more frequent' (Svetlik, 1992, p. 221).

For nurses in the former Yugoslavia, a central ethical challenge is to ensure that the particular experiences and needs of older people are recognized and addressed in a way that does not stereotype them as passive, dependent and pathetic creatures, but instead in one which respects their abilities and strengths and preserves their dignity. Achieving this, particularly in a situation where there are so many other priorities, is an extremely difficult task and requires well thought through arguments rather than emotive appeals. It requires that the different arguments for and against making distinctions are weighed up and the consequences of policies are evaluated. The question is not so much about ensuring the quality of services, but about ensuring that they are provided at all.

Conclusion

This chapter has tried to identify and explore some core ethical issues in the care of older people. These issues involve the distinction and differentiation between older people and others in society. The ethical issues which arise from making these distinctions are complex and they can lead either to stereotypes and ageism, or to a more sensitive understanding of the particular experiences of older people. The ethical and moral impact of making distinctions has to be seen against a range of political and policy contexts and examples have been drawn from three European countries where these contexts appear to be very different and where the central ethical issues facing nurses become subtly, or not so subtly, different. Where the political context is humanitarian, there is no dispute about access to services; instead, the focus is about quality of services and issues of choice, autonomy and empowerment. Where the political context is concerned with cost containment, the nursing task is to try to ensure that access to services is maintained and that provision is at least adequate. Where the political context does not firmly identify older people as a specific group, the nursing task is to ensure that the situations in which older people find themselves, and the problems that they face, are made apparent to others. This can be illustrated by Figure 10.1.

All of these ethical tasks involve some form of advocacy, either by articulating the needs of older people or by empowering them to direct service provision by articulating their needs

Formulation	Ethical task
Humanitarian formulation	Ensuring quality of services
Organizational formulation	Ensuring access to services
No formulation	Exploring and communicating the needs of older people, so that services can be provided

Figure 10.1   Formulations of the problems of old age and their associated ethical tasks

themselves. This advocacy, however, needs to take many things into account: the ageism inherent in so many cultures; the imbalance of power between professional and client; the reluctance of some older people to voice their wishes; and the ever-present danger of marshalling public support through appeals to pity which demean older people and reduce them to passive recipients of care. There is also some degree of hierarchical structure in these tasks. Where the political context is primitive, as in the case where the needs of older people have not been formulated, then the corresponding ethical tasks are very basic and are about establishing the need for care. Where the political context is more sophisticated, then the ethical tasks are qualitatively different and are about issues of access and quality in care. What is central to all of these ethical tasks, however, is that nurses take a wider view of ethical issues and see them not only as part of the day-to-day business of giving care, but as being inextricably linked to the political and policy contexts in which care is given.

References

Abrahamson, P. (1991) 'Welfare for the elderly in Denmark: from institutionalisation to self-reliance', *Eurosocial Report*, **40**(2): 35–61.

Arber, S. and Ginn, J. (1991) *Gender and Later Life: A Sociological Analysis of Resources and Constraints*. (London: Sage).

Armstrong, D. (1983) 'The fabrication of nurse–patient relationships', *Social Science and Medicine*, **17**(8): 457–60.

Baker, D.E. (1983) 'Care in the geriatric ward: an account of two styles of nursing', in Wilson-Barnet, J. (ed.) *Nursing Research: Ten Studies in Patient Care*. (John Wiley & Sons: Chichester), pp. 101–17.

Becker, L.C. (1986) *Reciprocity*. (Routledge: London).

Beveridge, W. (1942) *Social Insurance and Allied Services*, Cmnd 6404. (HMSO: London).

Binstock, R. (1984) 'Reframing the agenda of politics on ageing', in Minkler, M. and Stes, C. (eds) *Readings in the Political Economy of Ageing*. (Farmingdale: Baywood, New York), pp. 199–212.

Blaikie, A. (1994) 'Ageing and consumer culture: will we reap the whirlwind?', *Generations Review*, **4**(4): 5–7.

Boyajian, J.A. (1988) 'On reaching a new agenda: self-determination and ageing', in Thornton, J.E. and Winkler, E.R. (eds) *Ethics and Ageing*. (University of British Columbia Press: Vancouver), pp. 16–30.

Evers, H.K. (1981) 'The creation of patient carers in geriatric wards; aspects of policy and practice', *Social Science and Medicine*, **15**(1): 581–8.

Giarchi, G.G. (1996) *Caring for Older Europeans: Comparative Studies in 29 Countries*. (Arena: Aldershot).

Ginn, J. (1993) 'Grey power: age-based organisations' response to structured inequalities', *Critical Social Policy*, **13**(2): 23–47.

Hugman, R. (1996) 'Policies for the care of older people in Europe', *Health Care in Later Life*, **1**(4): 211–21.

Jamieson, A. (1990) 'Informal care in Europe' in Jamieson, A. and Illsley, R. (eds) *Contrasting European Policies for the Care of Older People*. (Avebury: Aldershot), pp. 3–21.

Johansen, L.N. (1986) 'Denmark', in Flora, P. (ed.) *Growth to Limits: the Western European States since World War Two*, vol. 1. (Walter de Gruyter: Berlin), pp. 293–381.

Kendrick, K.D. (1997) 'Advocacy in later life: an ethical analysis', *Health Care in Later Life*, **2**(1): 253–60.

Longmate, N. (1974) *The Workhouse*. (Temple Smith: London).

Macintyre, S. (1977) 'Old age as a social problem', in Dingwall, R., Health, C., Reid, M. and Stacey, M. (eds) *Health Care and Health Knowledge*. (Croom Helm: London), pp. 39–64.

Menzies, I. (1960) *The Functioning of Social Systems as a Defence against Anxiety*. (Tavistock: London).

Milosavljevic, M. and Ruzica, M. (1989) 'Yugoslavia – the effects of the economic and political crisis', in Munday, B. (ed.) *The Crisis in Welfare: An International Perspective on Social Services and Social Work*. (Harvester Wheatsheaf: London), pp. 155–80.

Norman, A. (1987) *Aspects of Ageism: A Discussion Paper*. (Centre for Policy on Ageing: London).

Ramhoej, N.E. (1992) 'Denmark', in Munday, B. (ed.) *Social Services in the Member States of the European Community: A Handbook of Information and Data*. (University of Kent: Canterbury), pp. 1–33.

Reed, J. (1989) 'All dressed up and nowhere to go: nursing assessment in geriatric wards', unpublished PhD thesis, University of Northumbria: Newcastle.

Reed, J. and Ground, I. (1996) *Philosophy for Nursing*. (Edward Arnold: London).

Ruzica, M., Hojnik-Zupanc, I. and Svetlik, I. (1991) 'Yugoslavia', in Evers H.K. and Svetlik, I. (eds) *New Welfare Mixes in Care for the Elderly*, vol. 1. (European Centre for Social Welfare Policy and Research: Vienna), pp. 73–93.

Seedhouse, D. (1988) *Ethics: The Heart of Health Care*. (John Wiley & Sons: London).

Svetlik, I. (1992) 'The future for welfare pluralism in Yugoslavia', in Deacon, B. (ed.) *Social Policy, Social Justice and Citizenship in Eastern Europe*. (Avebury: Aldershot), pp. 211–77.

Till, R. (1993) 'Ageing in literature', in Kaim-Caudle, P., Keithley, J. and Mullender, A. (eds) *Aspects of Ageing: A Celebration of the European Year of Older People and Solidarity between Generations*. (Whiting & Birch: London), pp. 140–7.

Troyansky, D. (1996) 'Progress report: the history of old age in the western world', *Ageing and Society*, **16**: 233–43.

Vincent, J. and Mudrovcic, Z. (1993) 'Lifestyles and perceptions of elderly people and old age in Bosnia and Herzegovina', in Arber, S. and Evandrou, M. (eds) *Ageing, Independence and the Life Course*. (Jessica Kingsley: London), pp. 90–105.

Walker, A. (1993) 'Older people in Europe: perceptions and realities', in Kaim-Caudle, P., Keithley, J. and Mullender, A. (eds) *Aspects of Ageing: A Celebration of the European Year of Older People and Solidarity between Generations*. (Whiting & Birch: London), pp. 8–24.

Wilderom, C. (in collaboration with Gottschalk, G.) (1991) 'Denmark', in Nijkamp, P., Pacolet, J., Spinnewyn, H., Vollering, A., Wilderom, C. and Winters, S. (eds) *Services for the Elderly in Europe: A Cross-national Comparative Study*, 2nd edn. (Commission of the European Communities: Brussels), pp. 113–33.

Suggestions for further reading

Bytheway, B. (1995) *Ageism*. (Open University: Buckinghamshire).

Hugman, R. (1994) *Ageing and the Care of Older People in Europe*. (St Martin's Press: New York).

Thornton, J.E. and Winkler, E.R. (1988) *Ethics and Ageing*. (University of British Columbia Press: Vancouver).

11

Ethical Issues in Critical Care Nursing

Kevin David Kendrick

Introduction

The thrust of this chapter is to explore research findings about issues that cause ethical concern for critical care nurses in Europe. Comparisons between the experience of critical care nurses in Sweden and the United Kingdom will be made for the simple reason that these are the only two European countries that have, to date, published research papers related to the way that nurses deal with, or feel about, the moral dimensions of critical care practice. The first stage in this process will be to explore the preparation of critical care nurses to deal with ethical issues and to identify the nature and essence of nursing ethics in relation to the delivery of critical care.

Ethics: a common concern

Recent decades have seen major scientific and technological advances in the care of critically ill patients. Conditions that once would almost certainly have caused death are now confronted by a broad range of complex interventions (Margotta, 1996). The essential elements in this type of care delivery and management may be defined as follows:

> Critical care is optimally delivered to patients by a team of highly trained personnel who are provided with the physical facilities,

equipment and organisational structures that will enable them to fulfil their life-saving and life-preserving function and to do so effectively and efficiently. The intensive care unit has therefore been looked on as the 'hospital's hospital' (Noc and Weil, 1996, p.3).

Meeting and dealing with situations that have an ethical dimension is an intrinsic part of working in this sort of demanding environment and such situations always create a challenge to those involved with them. Facing difficult moral scenarios can cause doubt, anxiety and turbulence among those working in critical care areas and can also contribute to staff burn-out and high turnover (Fenton, 1988; Kendrick and Cubbin, 1996).

To some extent, education is culpable for this situation as it has been slow to offer critical care nurses the opportunities to engage with the 'tools' of ethical analysis (Melia, 1996). This deficiency was largely the result of the cursory attention paid to the place of ethics in post-basic courses in critical care; an omission that has only recently been revisited and addressed (Kendrick, 1994a; Leavitt, 1996). Thus, although nurses across the European Community are drenched with educational opportunities leading to technical competence and, ultimately, expertise (Timmermann, 1996), their ability to engage with the moral demands of critical care delivery has traditionally been left wanting. This is a point upon which some commentators have cogently commented: 'what is technical competence worth when shackled by moral incompetence?' (Hunt, 1991, cited in Tschudin and Marks-Maran, 1993, p. 77).

Summarizing these themes, it can be said that European critical care nurses are faced with the moral dilemmas involved in working in an environment that is technologically advanced. However, there is little educational or practical support to help them confront and frame ethical concerns which can lead to angst, disillusionment and low morale (Bertolini, 1994).

Beyond medical ethics

Many of the published papers dealing with the moral concerns associated with critical care have traditionally been subsumed under the umbrella term 'medical ethics'. The following list high-lights some of the subjects that frequently arise in the literature:

- The ethics of organ transplantation (Blackwell, 1989; Anaise *et al.*, 1990)
- Considerations of age and the allocation of medical resources (Levine, 1989; Dimingo, 1993)
- Do not resuscitate orders in intensive care (Bedell, 1986; Brown, 1990; Marsden, 1993)
- Brain stem death (Pallis, 1983).

There is no doubt that these subjects have moral relevance, especially to doctors and nurses. Seedhouse (1988, p. 34) refers to such dilemmas as 'specific or dramatic ethics' and argues that such scenarios are usually characterized by a pressing need to make a clear decision about a definite course of action. To illuminate his position, he gives the following example:

> For instance, the choice might be whether to switch off a life support machine in order to transplant a variety of organs to three waiting recipients, all of whom stand a good chance of further fulfilling life, or whether to keep the machine on because of the slim possibility that the body might regain consciousness (Seedhouse, 1988, p. 34).

Such dilemmas are usually categorized as 'medical ethics' because it is the doctor who has the clinical and legal autonomy to be prescriptive about the chosen outcome. To try and increase nursing's autonomy and continued professional emergence, nurses in some countries increasingly undertake work that was once performed only by doctors (Marshall, 1997). In effect, this has challenged and blurred traditional working bound-aries and in the United Kingdom, this situation has been formal-ized by nursing's governing body in its document *The Scope of Professional Practice* (UKCC, 1992).

In essence, this document sought to broaden the parameters of professional autonomy by encouraging nurses to deliver safe, competent and accountable care. It gave nurses the freedom to perform activities that fully challenged their skills and expertise, while at the same time achieving a corresponding reduction in the working hours of junior doctors.

Some commentators have explored nursing's preoccupation with increased levels of technical care giving as Castledine (1993, p. 686) suggests:

> I do not mean to imply that the nurse of tomorrow should take on all the tasks that doctors do not want to perform. Rather, I am suggesting that the present and future role of nurses covers a wide span, ranging from the most simple tasks to the expert, professional techniques that are necessary in acute life-threatening situations.

A key supporting theme is that professional autonomy increases through such avenues, as it may be argued that if the technical delivery of care is increasingly shared between doctors and nurses, they should, at the very least, have equal voice when decisions are ethically sensitive. To do less than this denies the moral agency of the nurse.

Such notions are, however, fallacious because they create an illusion that nursing's increased involvement with technical care somehow increases the worth and currency of the ethical decisions made by its practitioners. This form of argument is similar to the common misnomer that increased technical competence somehow increases the essence of nursing's value and professional creed. Instead, the worth of the nurse as a moral agent is intrinsic and advancing technical ability does not add to this. The nub of the issue is captured by Bergum (1994, p. 78):

> The nurse and the doctor must move from the technological reasoning of the scientific laboratory to the bedside, where tact and thoughtfulness may bring forth new and necessary knowledge. The startling picture of real people being fragmented into abstract parts can be lessened through further development of abilities to enter relationships with patients that focus on understanding human experience.

Sharing ethical decision-making

Difficult ethical decisions should be explored on a shared footing that values each practitioner's right to voice his or her moral concerns and perspective, be they nurse, doctor or other member of the team. Such themes are essentially Kantian and reflect the third formulation of the Categorical Imperative which states: 'in wishing to be moral, individuals must act as members of a community where everybody is seen as having intrinsic worth (ends in their own right)' (Korner, 1982, p. 63). Commenting on this formulation of the Categorical Imperative, Kendrick (1993, p. 924) applied its sentiment to nursing practice and states:

> As nurses, we often meet colleagues or clients who hold differing views to our own. While it is legitimate to hold contradicting attitudes towards the same issue, the central principle is that both parties have equal licence to hold, express and defend their respective positions.

Doctors have no mandate to hold sway over moral decisions which should be based on a shared governance. If the current vogue for interdisciplinary working and learning is to be founded on more than rhetoric and empty semantics, it must grasp the ethos of 'teamwork' in its fullest sense and meaning. In this way, the central ethical issues that face nurses in critical care are no different from those faced by colleagues in other areas of care delivery. The context may be different, but the desire to be acknowledged and listened to remains the same. The common essence, focus and purpose of nursing surpasses contextual considerations and it is this that creates and defines its moral milieu. Taking this further, Melia (1996, p. 141) states:

> At heart then, all these issues come back to the same principles that nursing in general relies on in order to focus on its moral basis. We do not need to create a special ethics for intensive care, what we work with already in nursing will suffice, it is only the cases and contexts that differ, the principles transcend the setting.

What is certain is that ethics is a vital, challenging and vibrant part of nurses' itinerary; as Tschudin (1993, p. 1) eloquently asserts: 'Ethics is not only at the heart of nursing, it is the heart of nursing.' With ethics firmly placed at the centre of the nursing endeavour, we will now consider specific research that explores how nurses deal with the moral dimensions of delivering critical care.

The Swedish experience

In a major Swedish study, Söderberg and Norberg (1993) conducted research into situations that caused ethical difficulty in delivering intensive care. This involved 20 doctors, 20 registered nurses and 20 enrolled nurses, each narrating their experiences about situations that had caused them moral concern. The main reason the researchers chose this approach was because 'narratives about ethically difficult care situations may disclose differences of perceptions, feelings, reasoning and actions' (p. 2008).

Each narrated story was recorded and later transcribed. Each transcript was then examined using phenomenological–hermeneutic analysis (Ricoeur, 1976, 1984). This involved initially dividing the plot of each story according to the dominant influence of one of two themes: action ethics or relational ethics. In this respect, Söderberg and Norberg adopted Lindseth's (1982) distinction that action ethics is concerned with focusing on the right choice of action within the limitations of a given context and situation, while relational ethics is concerned with how people relate to each other in various situations.

During the structural analysis the main context of each story was characterized according to whether an action element or a relational element dominated. In order to establish which perspective was dominant in respective stories, the researchers asked the following questions:

- What choice of action does the story represent? (action ethics)
- What does the story tell us about the relationships between the actors? (relational ethics)

Perhaps the most pertinent theme emerging from this research was the finding that physicians, registered nurses and enrolled nurses all 'saw themselves as equally lacking in influence in ethically difficult care situations' (p. 2008). This finding makes a fascinating basis for comparison as we explore research that reflects the experiences of nurses in a British intensive care unit.

The British experience

In a small-scale, published research study, Basset (1995) used a phenomenological framework to explore how intensive care nurses deal with ethical dilemmas. He describes the purpose and focus of the project in the following way:

> The researcher in carrying out this research does not expect to gain an absolute 'factual truth', but hopes to gain 'insight' into this key area. From this he hopes to better manage his own approach to the ethical decision making process and by dissemination of the findings, aid others in considering their own positions (p. 168).

Basset asked four nurses to take part in a guided discussion, which would be recorded, subsequently transcribed and analysed. Throughout the discussion, the researcher used open-ended questions to guide the dialogue. The recorded discussion took place in a small private room and lasted for an hour and 15 minutes. When analysing the transcript of the discussion, Basset divided the statements into categories and then into themes. In describing this process he states:

> A knowledge of intensive care nursing proved to be useful in this process, understanding the language of intensive care nurses. Statements and phrases directly relating to ethical factors were highlighted and bracketed, this process helping to maintain reliability and validity by reducing possible bias (p. 168).

Three themes emerged from the analysis: senselessness, stress and impotence. To reflect the theme of senselessness, Basset quotes the feelings of one nurse involved in the care of a patient whose life was seemingly being prolonged beyond any chance of recovery:

> I remember a patient who was quite literally 'rotting' and in a terrible state, but we (as nurses) had to keep this patient as comfortable as possible. This went on for several days, there was no chance of recovery (p. 166).

The theme of stress is illustrated by a nurse talking about the sometimes futile purpose of ventilation: 'sometimes you go off duty and the patient just goes with you, it is impossible sometimes to forget them (the patient). You just keep thinking about the stupidity of keeping them ventilated at any cost' (p. 166).

The final theme, impotence, finds most focus in the nurses' feelings about relationships with doctors: 'I consider myself and my colleagues as being expert in what we do, we are as least as professionally well qualified as many doctors, but we are not considered as such by some' (p. 166).

Basset acknowledges that the transcribed material concentrates on the negative; however, he also argues that the key aim was to encourage nurses to talk about the ethical issues that cause distress within the unit. The final comment in his paper holds tremendous resonance for nurses working in intensive care units: 'It is important that we as nurses involved in critical care learn more about ethics, value conflicts and communication. The dilemmas we face will not disappear, there will be more and more in the future' (p. 169).

Comparisons and reasons

It is interesting that Söderberg and Norberg's Swedish research showed doctors and nurses to feel 'equally lacking in influence' with regards to moral decision-making; conversely, Basset's British research found that nurses often felt ethically impotent because they considered that doctors held a demeaning attitude towards them. Such themes are further supported by Johnstone (1989, p. 1) who states:

> Some doctors apparently believe that nurses are incapable of sound rational thought, and are incapable of grasping the essence of sound moral thinking. These doctors are loath to accept that nurses have any independent moral responsibility when caring for patients. As these doctors are invariably in positions of power, they are more than able to ensure that a nursing perspective on patient care, and related moral issues, are effectively constrained.

Part of the reason Swedish nurses and doctors felt equally fettered with regards to moral decision-making may lie in the absence of status, class, gender and other social barriers. Such themes have traditionally enmeshed and supported restrictive working practices and unequal opportunities in the British social system.

The British health care system is a microcosm of its broader social milieu and reflects its dominant norms, values and means of maintaining the status quo. Such themes are further supported by the experience of foreign nurses who come to work in the United Kingdom. Unshackled by the restrictive elements of power and status so inherent in British society, they do not acquiesce to the dominance of medical patriarchy. Instead as Mackay (1993, p. 122) asserts:

> These overseas nurses may show none of the deference and acqui-escence of the British trained nurse. They are not part of the class and status system. Because of that, these nurses are treated differ-ently, enjoying more of an equal status with the medical profes-sion; and they treat doctors differently, as equals. These nurses can be particularly scathing about home grown nurses' refusal to ques-tion doctor's decisions or to take responsibility.

However, despite this level of perceived authority by foreign nurses working in the United Kingdom, the reality is that, with regard to diagnosis and treatment, nurses are powerless and must await the legal prerequisite of 'doctors' orders' before implementing the care associated with such orders. Once again, the cure-orientated aspects of clinical medicine seem to hold more intrinsic worth than those of nursing's care-based elements. This is a theme which continues to influence the hidden agenda in nurse–doctor relationships. While this perception is allowed to continue there is little chance of an enacted sense of parity between doctors and nurses. Adshead and Dickenson (1993, p. 167) reflect these sentiments in the following way:

> If nursing is defined as being about caring, and medicine about curing, medicine will continue to be seen as more important. If the role of the female paradigm profession of nursing is seen as caring, the old stereotype of the nurse as the doctor's 'helpmeet' will be revived. Caring is likely to be seen as less important than curing because we fear death and wrongly attribute to medicine the power to cure us of mortality.

This section has suggested and explored some possible reasons to explain the differences towards ethical decision-making between doctors and nurses in Sweden and Britain. What has emerged is that British nurses are submerged in a power-based scenario that perpetuates and reifies the mythical theme of medicine's hold over death. Giving this further credence, interprofessional relationships take place in a working culture that fully mirrors the British class system in which issues of gender, educational background and status are important influences.

Given the combination of factors that maintain and reinforce nursing's subservient position to medicine, it is not surprising to find British nurses playing such a small role in ethical decision-making. This feature not only disempowers nurses but chisels away at a concept that is central to nursing's professional creed, that of patient advocacy. Logically, if research suggests that British critical care nurses have little say in clinical situations that are morally problematic, how can they play an effective role as patient advocates? That this role assumes such central importance for critical care nurses is evidenced by the fact that patients requiring critical care are frequently unable to speak for themselves due to the nature of their conditions. To explore this question demands further analysis of those themes that surround advocacy in the delivery of critical care.

Ethical advocacy

In recent decades, the mantle of advocacy, with its central purpose of representing, safeguarding and promoting the interests of patients, has been firmly grasped by the nursing profession. One result from this has been a host of papers arguing that nurses are ideally placed to play an advocatory role (Abrahams, 1978; Murphy and Hunter, 1984; Penn, 1994) as it represents a key element in the ethos of caring. Advocacy presents itself when practitioners become an 'active voice' when, for whatever reason, patients feel unable to articulate or represent their own best interests. Such notions seem to reflect the core moral principles of beneficence, non-maleficence and respect for persons. Indeed, the *Concise Oxford Dictionary* (1992, p. 18) reinforces such themes with its definition of an advocate as a person 'who pleads for another'.

Against this background, advocacy is portrayed as a virtuous endeavour that sits comfortably with the values that have traditionally underpinned contemporary Western health care. The essence of the nurse's role as patient advocate in critical care is given sharp focus by Drought and Liaschenko (1995, p. 297) who state, 'Nursing's role is to hold foremost the overall well-being of the patient, and to advocate for the patient, not for the technology'.

Developing the notion of advocacy in critical care even further, Rushton (1995, p. 388) states:

> The goal of advocacy is to enable the patient, family and significant others to adjust to the changes in their own unique way. Nursing actions are directed toward maximising the control exerted by the patient and family, and assisting them to find unique meaning or purpose in their living or their dying and to realise goals that promote a meaningful life or death.

It is interesting to note that much of the interplay concerning advocacy involves the nurse playing an intercessory role between the patient and the doctor. A transactional analysis of the relationships between doctors, nurses and patients would certainly suggest an imbalance of power between these key players, as Chadwick and Tadd (1992, p. 65) state: 'characteristically the doctor has been portrayed as "all knowing" and powerful; the nurse as caring, unselfish, obedient and submissive; and the patient as helpless and utterly trusting'.

This triad of professional relationships discussed by Chadwick and Tadd is often placed under the umbrella term of 'parentalism' and results in the patient being treated in a way that is directly analogous to that of a child; reflecting the essence of this concept, Kendrick (1995, p. 241) states:

> The characteristics of parentalism are heavily imprinted upon the traditional picture of the relationship between doctors, nurses and their patients. Resulting from this image of the 'pseudo-family' is a completely disempowered patient who passively conforms to the dominant wishes of 'mother' and 'father'.

Given what has been said about the lack of power that nurses hold in ethical decision-making, the language of advocacy pales into rhetoric, especially when viewed against the realities of nurses' experience as documented in research (Mackay, 1993; Basset, 1995; Kendrick and Cubbin, 1996). Well-meaning, but quite empty, semantics abound in nursing literature and a further example is given by Brown (1985, p. 26) who states that advocacy is a 'means of transferring power back to the patient'. Given the lack of power nurses have in their relationships with doctors, how can such idealistic terms become reality? Put another way, how can the disempowered nurse empower the disempowered patient? In the light of such themes it is questionable whether nurses have a sufficient base to act as patient advocates and this finds particular focus when examining the notion of 'best interests' and who defines them.

Defining best interests – who decides?

At the core of advocacy lies the notion of 'best interests'. Murphy and Hunter (1984, p. 24) translate this to the delivery of patient care:

> The professional, while obligated to act in the patient's best interests, is not permitted to define that interest in any way contrary to the patient's definition; it is not the professional but the patient that shall define what 'best interests' shall mean.

Relating these themes to clinical reality reveals a split between well-placed rhetoric and power-based reality. We have already noted that nurses share an unequal power base with doctors and these damaging but influential themes reflect negatively on the value of nursing and nurses. This is further supported and reinforced by media representations. Taking this further, Mackay (1989, p. 46) points out that:

> Stereotypes in the mass media appear to enhance the status of doctors at the expense of nurses. Nurses are presented in the media as less helpful and less empathetic to the needs of patients and doctors. Yet when the reality of nurses' work is considered the stereotype is revealed for what it is: a put down of nurses and of women.

Thus, a structural analysis of advocacy reveals a scenario that is supposed to empower a disempowered patient; however, the previous reference strongly indicates that nurses are also victims in a health care equation based upon power. To a large extent, nurses have been authors of their own oppression and traditionally have done little to confront the level of disparity between themselves and doctors at an operational level. Exploring reasons for this, Kendrick (1994b, p. 78) argues:

> Nursing's failure to divorce itself successfully and universally from the medical model as a *modus operandi* for the delivery of care must be seen as a major contributing factor to the subordinate position nursing holds in relation to medicine.

Against this backdrop, the notion of the nurse as the patient's advocate seems fairly ineffectual. It is also unlikely that patients will be able to define their own 'best interests' when they hold least power in a power-based system. With analytical verve, Allmark and Klarzynski (1992, p. 34) comment upon the dubious nature of patient advocacy:

> An advocate should plead someone's cause as the person, and not the advocate, sees it. If a liberal lawyer pleads the cause of a neo-Nazi group to have freedom of speech then this is true advocacy. A nurse is unable to provide the alcoholic with a drink, plead for the overdose not to be treated, and for the sectioned patient to be allowed to leave.

Relating the thrust of Allmark and Klarzynski's argument to critical care, how many nurses have the autonomy and power to stop treatment when clinical indicators point towards the futility of continuance, for example in the case where a patient has total organ failure? This is clearly mirrored by revisiting the words of one nurse in Basset's research: 'I remember a patient who was quite literally 'rotting' and in a terrible state, but we (as nurses) had to keep this patient as comfortable as possible. This went on for several days, there was no chance of recovery' (1995, p. 166).

How does the notion of the nurse as patient advocate stand in the light of such a damning remark? Clearly, advocacy is a power-laden concept that instrumentally supports a hierarchical structure which threatens patient autonomy, choice and, ulti-mately, dignity. Reflecting these themes further, Allmark and Klarzynski (1992, p. 35) make the following comment: 'To suggest that a patient has an advocate when it is that very person who may be involved in the treatment that the patient is trying to resist is analogous to suggesting that the police can act as advocates for people in custody.'

Conclusion

This chapter has explored some of the key themes that influence and direct critical care nurses in relation to the moral dimensions of their practice. In comparing findings between two European countries where research has been conducted, Swedish nurses were found to be on an equal footing with doctors in relation to moral decision-making, in that both groups felt 'equally lacking in influence'. This compared favourably with British findings where the key themes of sense-lessness, stress and impotence framed the disempowered position that critical care nurses experience in moral decision-making alongside doctors. While this impoverished state is maintained, key elements at the heart of nursing's professional creed will be challenged and neutralized. This chapter has explored this notion in relation to patient advocacy.

What has emerged from this exercise is an understanding that ethics is fundamental to the work of practitioners, be they doctors, nurses or any other member of the 'hands-on' team. In Sweden, the very fact that nurses and doctors felt 'equally lacking' strongly supports the need for an educational programme that equips practitioners with the ethical 'tools' to confront the moral dimensions of their work. Scandinavia has a strong background in shared professional learning and ethics would fit comfortably into this policy (Regional Health University, 1981).

In the UK, doctors must stop seeing situations that are ethically relevant as something to be subsumed under the broad notion of a 'clinical decision'. In essence, this should mean shared governance with other practitioners, as ethics belongs to us all and is not solely the domain of medicine. Educational programmes that are clinically relevant and delivered in or near to the clinical setting are ideal avenues for bringing team members together to explore the ethical issues pertinent to critical care. Cogently reflecting these themes, Melia (1996, p. 138) provides the perfect focus for such an endeavour:

Intensive care, with its emphasis on team work, is an ideal setting in which to promote health care ethics as a multi-disciplinary enterprise rather than as a major arena in which to battle out medical versus nursing ethics.

The gauntlet has been thrown down, who among us will pick it up?

References

Abrahams, N.A. (1978) 'A contrary view of the nurse as patient advocate', *Nursing Forum*, **17**(1): 260–6.

Adshead, G. and Dickenson, D. (1993) 'Why do doctors and nurses disagree?', in Dickensen, D. and Johnson, M. (eds) *Death, Dying and Bereavement.* (Sage: London), pp. 161–8.

Allmark, P. and Klarzynski, R. (1992) 'The case against nurse advocacy', *British Journal of Nursing*, **2**: 133–6.

Anaise, D., Smith, R., Ishimaru, M. *et al.* (1990) 'An approach to organ salvage from non-heartbeating cadaver donors under existing legal and ethical requirements', *Transplantation*, **49**(3): 290–4.

Basset, C. (1995) 'Critical care nurses: ethical dilemmas, a phenomenological approach', *Care of the Critically Ill*, **11**:166–9.

Bedell, S.E. (1986) 'Do-Not-Resuscitate orders for critically ill patients in the hospital: how are they used and what is their impact?', *Journal of the American Medical Association*, **256**(4): 233–7.

Bergum, V. (1994) 'Knowledge for ethical care', *International Journal of Nursing Ethics*, **1**(2): 71–9.

Bertolini, C.L. (1994) 'Ethical decision-making in intensive care: a nurse's perspective', *Intensive and Critical Care Nursing*, **10**(1): 58–63.

Blackwell, C. (1989) 'Elective ventilation for transplant purposes', *Intensive and Critical Care Nursing*, **9**(2): 122–8.

Brown, C. (1990) 'Limiting care: is CPR for everyone?', *Clinical Issues in Critical Care*, **1**(16): 1–68.

Brown, M. (1985) 'Matter of commitment', *Nursing Times*, **81**(18): 26–7.

Castledine, G. (1993) 'Nurses should welcome a wider scope of practice', *British Journal of Nursing*, **2**(13): 686–7.

Chadwick, R. and Tadd, W. (1992) *Ethics and Nursing Practice: A Case Study Approach.* (Macmillan: Basingstoke).

Concise Oxford Dictionary (1992) (Oxford University Press: Oxford).

Dimingo, J. (1993) 'Commentary on mortality in intensive care patients with respiratory disease: is age important?', *Nursing Scan in Critical Care Nursing*, **3**(1): 8–11.

Drought, T.S. and Liaschenko, J. (1995) 'Ethical practice in a technological age', *Critical Care Nursing Clinics of North America*, **7**: 7227–303.

Fenton, M. (1988) 'Moral distress in clinical practice: implications for the nurse administrator', *Canadian Journal of Nursing Administration*, **1**(3): 8–11.

Hunt, G. (1991) 'The concept of moral responsibility', Paper presented at the Inaugural Conference of the National Centre for Nursing and Midwifery Ethics, Queen Charlotte College, Thames Valley University, cited in: Tschudin, V. and Marks-Maran, D. (eds) 1993) *Ethics: A Primer for Nurses: Workshop Guide*. (Baillière Tindall: London).

Johnstone, M.J. (1989) *Bioethics: A Nursing Perspective*. (Baillière Tindall: Sydney).

Kendrick, K. (1993) 'Understanding ethics in nursing practice', *British Journal of Nursing*, **2**(18): 920–5.

Kendrick, K. (1994a) 'Building bridges: teaching ward-based ethics', *International Journal of Nursing Ethics*, **1**(1): 35–41.

Kendrick, K. (1994b) 'Towards professional parity', *International Journal of Reviews in Clinical Gerontology*, **4**(4): 277–9.

Kendrick, K. (1995) 'Ethical pathways in cancer and palliative care', in David, J. (ed.) *Cancer Care: Prevention, Treatment and Palliation*. (Chapman & Hall: London), pp. 224–44.

Kendrick, K. and Cubbin, B. (1996) 'Ethics in the intensive care unit: a need for research', *International Journal of Nursing Ethics*, **3**(3): 157–64.

Korner, S. (1982) *Kant*. (Penguin: Harmondsworth).

Leavitt, F.J. (1996) 'Educating nurses for their future role in bioethics', *International Journal of Nursing Ethics*, **3**(1): 39–52.

Levine, M.E. (1989) 'Ration or rescue: the elderly person in critical care', *Critical Care Nursing Quarterly*, **12**(1): 82–9.

Lindseth, A. (1982) 'The role of caring in nursing ethics', in Oden, G. (ed.) *Quality Development in Nursing Care: From Practice to Science*. (Linkoping Collaborating Centre: Linkoping), pp. 68–78.

Mackay, L. (1989) *Nursing A Problem*. (Open University Press: Milton Keynes).

Mackay, L. (1993) *Conflict in Care: Medicine and Nursing*. (Chapman & Hall: London).

Margotta, R. (1996) *The History of Medicine*. (Hamlyn: London).

Marsden, C. (1993) '"Do not resuscitate" orders and end of life care planning', *American Journal of Critical Care*, **1**(1): 1770–9.

Marshall, J. (1997) 'Protocols and emergency nurse practitioners', *Nursing Times*, **93**(14): 58–9.

Melia, K. (1996) 'The nursing perspective', in Pace, A, and McLean, S.A.M. (eds) *Ethics and Law in Intensive Care*. (Oxford University Press: Oxford), pp. 134–41.

Murphy, C. and Hunter, H. (1994) *Ethical Problems in the Nurse–Patient Relationship.* (Allwin & Bacon: Boston).

Noc, M. and Weil, M.H. (1996) 'Critical care', in Tinker, J., Browne, D.R.G. and Sibbald, W.J. (eds) *Critical Care: Standards, Audit and Ethics.* (Edward Arnold: London), pp. 3–10.

Pallis, C. (1983) *ABC of Brainstem Death.* (British Medical Association: London).

Penn, K. (1994) 'Patient advocacy in palliative care', *British Journal of Nursing*, **3**(1): 40–2.

Regional Health University Proposal for a trial project in Ostergotland (LIV) (1981) Report from the Linkoping Commission on Integrated Health Care Education, Regional Health University: Linkoping.

Ricoeur, P. (1976) *Interpretation Theory: Discourse and the Surplus of Meaning.* (Texas Christian University Press: Fort Worth, Tex.).

Ricoeur, P. (1984) The model of the text: meaningful action considered as text', *Journal of Social Research*, **51**: 185–218.

Rushton, C.H. (1995) 'Creating an ethical practice environment: a focus on advocacy', *Critical Care Nursings Clinics of North America*, **7**(2): 387–97.

Seedhouse, D. (1988) *Ethics; The Heart of Health Care.* (John Wiley & Sons: Chichester).

Söderberg, A. and Norberg, A. (1993) 'Intensive care: situations of ethical difficulty', *Journal of Advanced Nursing*, **18**: 2008–14.

Timmermann, A.M. (1996) 'Intensive care: nursing, staffing and training in the EC', in Tinker, J., Browne, D.R.G. and Sibbald, W.J. (eds) *Critical Care: Standards, Audit and Ethics.* (Edward Arnold: London), pp. 212–22.

UKCC (United Kingdom Central Council for Nursing, Midwifery and Health Visiting) (1992) *The Scope of Professional Practice.* (UKCC: London).

Suggestions for further reading

Braine, D. and Lesser, H. (1988) *Ethics, Technology and Medicine.* (Avebury: Aldershot).

Lee, R. and Morgan, D. (eds) (1994) *Law and Ethics at the End of Life.* (Routledge: London).

Pace, A. and McLean, S.A.M. (eds) (1996) *Ethics and Law in Intensive Care.* (Oxford University Press: Oxford).

Tinker, J., Browne, D.R.G. and Sibbald, W.J. (eds) (1996) *Critical Care: Standards, Audit and Ethics.* (Edward Arnold: London).

Tuxill, C. (1994) 'Ethical aspects of critical care', in Millar, B. and Burnard, P. (eds) *Critical Care Nursing: Caring for the Critically Ill Adult.* (Baillière Tindall: London), pp. 250–72.

12

Nursing Ethics at the End of Life

Verena Tschudin

Introduction

'Human beings should revere life and accept death' (Thiroux, 1995, p. 180). With this simple statement Thiroux sums up what he describes as the Principle of the Value of Life. Because death has taken the place of an enemy to be fought with every means possible it can be said that we do not show the reverence due to life either. Today's world demands more and more from life (meaning here all life, plants and animals included) and when these demands cannot be met, we feel angry and try still harder not to accept the limits imposed by something which we cannot control. Because it is difficult to accept death, we try to defeat it with an emphasis on health and well-being which can border on excess. The claim has been made that because we do not accept death, countries are being ruined economically. Or, as Callahan (1990, p. 254) puts it, our 'single-minded ambition to overcome mortality will generate misery and social distortion [and] will create a house, our society, in which we would not want to live'. The ideals of the market-place favour the individual, but these trends concern society. It is in this dichotomy between individual needs and societal possibilities that our greatest problems and our greatest challenges may well lie.

This chapter will address some of the issues raised by the ethical concerns at the end of life. In European countries the issues are fairly similar, except for the Netherlands. This is one of the countries which will be compared with the United Kingdom (UK), the other being Switzerland, but references will also be made to other European countries.

End of life

In the literature the expression 'end of life' is used in preference to 'dying' as it can cover more specific issues. It is also perhaps a less emotive term, although it may be questionable whether or not this is helpful.

Under the heading of end of life several different issues can be addressed:

- Neonatal critical care
- Brain stem death
- Persistent vegetative state
- Care of the dying
- Care in different settings: such as intensive care, hospital, community
- Organ transplantation
- Care of the sick elderly
- Euthanasia
- Advance directives and living wills
- Resuscitation.

The most pressing problems faced by nurses in end of life situations are generally:

- When patients and clients request no further treatment and this is not respected
- When doctors order treatments and nurses do not agree with the orders
- When patients and clients are not informed of their conditions and request information
- When adequate care is difficult because of the patient's condition (fungating wounds, multiple disease problems, mental as well as physical illness) or the nurses' inexperience.

Perhaps the most pressing problem, as is so often the case, is that of communication: between nurses and doctors; nurses and patients; doctors and patients; nurses and families; or patients and their families. Ethical problems are problems of fundamental right and wrong, but what is right and wrong needs to be understood, heard, expressed and respected, not simply prescribed or dismissed.

End of life issues in the UK

The debate about end of life issues in the UK has been dominated by several well-publicized cases in recent years:

- Tony Bland: a young man who was injured at the Hillsborough Stadium in 1989 and was in a persistent vegetative state (PVS) before he was allowed to die (Ellis, 1992)
- Laura Davies: a six-year-old child, who had a bowel and liver transplant in the UK, and then a six-organ transplant in the USA (Turner, 1993)
- Dr Nigel Cox: a hospital doctor who gave one of his patients an injection of potassium chloride to end her life after she had repeatedly asked that she should be helped to die (Castledine, 1994).

These three major events, and others amounting to the actual care given or not on the basis of 'value for money', have shaped the discussion in the UK in the last few years. The debate has been polarized into issues of euthanasia and who should receive treatment which is of debatable value given the limited resources. Perhaps the most striking outcome of all these problems and discussions is that no-one has been prosecuted for murder or killing and no professional has been removed from a register.

Neonatal care

The amendment of 1991 to the Abortion Act 1967 put the upper gestation limit for abortion for most reasons as the end of the 24th week (Paintin, 1991). Alongside this, 'neonatal intensive care is an area where "hi-tech" medicine has been remarkably successful. Advances in perinatal care have been accompanied by improved survival among infants born in the middle to late second trimester who were previously considered non-viable' (Gill, 1994, p. 448).

Therefore, 'treatment withheld on a 24-week gestation baby in the neonatal intensive care unit might constitute a felony, whereas therapeutic termination of pregnancy of a similar gestation fetus is now legal' (Gill, 1994, p. 450). The dilemma is whether or not to provide resuscitation. According to Gill (1994, p. 450) 'the decision to resuscitate depends upon the personal philosophy of the primary care physicians and other health professionals, with variable input from parents'. Grimley (1995) describes a baby born at 29 weeks, weighing 930 grams who needed maximum ventilatory support. His outlook was poor: he had

> a 95% chance of severe physical disability (spastic quadriplegia), learning disabilities and visual impairment. ...With modern technology at our disposal, we are better able to prolong and save the lives of babies who previously would have died. It follows, that we are also in a position to decide whether or not to continue treatment and, if not, how death will occur (Grimley, 1995, p. 42).

Whereas in the past such premature infants would have died, we now have to make decisions regarding their lives and their deaths. Too often in the past, the parents' wishes have been disregarded. Grimley (1995, p. 43) sees it as the responsibility of nurses 'to facilitate more understanding and to enable more than just token participation by parents in the decision-making process'. This demands a high level of communication, of counselling skills, of empathy, as well as knowledge of laws and policies.

Care of the dying

In the UK, care of the dying has been pioneered as a special category of care by Dame Cicely Saunders. As a qualified nurse, social worker and medical doctor she was in a unique position to understand the plight of patients who were dying. It is legitimate to claim that the care of the dying in the UK has been developed and led by nurses. According to Bycroft and Brown:

> our confidence (as nurses) to stand alongside dying patients, no matter what happens to them, depends on us having knowledge, skills and support in our effort to understand the patients' needs, and to respond to them. Broadly, these needs will be:
>
> 1. to receive support based on understanding of their task of adjusting to dying;
> 2. to be relieved of distressing physical symptoms;
> 3. to know that their family and friends are supported, and will continue to be after their death (1996, p. 420).

Bycroft and Brown describe in detail the psychological support which patients and families should receive. The physical symptoms experienced by dying patients consist mainly of pain and the fear of pain, but anorexia, dry mouth, constipation, nausea, vomiting, insomnia, dyspnoea, cough or oedema (Bycroft and Brown, 1996, p. 428), are all well known.

The care of the dying has often been seen as a quest for giving quality of life to patients in preference to quantity, or the quest for a cure (Hunt, 1993). The transition from a search for cure to maintaining a quality which is acceptable is the area of greatest ethical problems. According to a Working Party Report (Gormally, 1994, p. 91) 'the first requirement of good terminal care is that the dying patient should be treated as a person'. This implies that much talking, listening and discussing should take place. 'At some point you have to talk about the purpose of life. Futile treatment, which cannot restore the patient's health, is not worth doing' (Shamash, 1995, p. 15).

The difference here between care of the dying and care for patients who are unconscious, mentally ill, or in persistent vegetative state (PVS), is essentially who is mainly or primarily involved in decision-making: the patient or close family, legal guardians or significant others. Dying is not a private affair, and other people are always involved, even if this may be a nurse caring for a person who has no relatives. Because nurses invest more and more care when someone is dying, while doctors invest less and less, it is imperative that nurses should be consulted in any decisions regarding the care that is to be given.

Care of the dying cannot be considered without mentioning hospices. The *Directory of Hospice Services in the UK and Republic of Ireland* (Hospice Information Services, 1997) lists 223 units with 3253 beds, about 400 home care teams and 234 day care centres available for the care of the dying, for a total population of about 60 million people. Hospices have changed their role considerably since their inception. Today they not only provide both physical and psychological care for the patients, but they also provide support for families during the patients' illness and in bereavement. Additionally, hospices are

> taking on the role of educational and resource centres, accessed for education and training purposes and for advice and support on issues relating to palliative care, by medical and nursing colleagues who are caring for patients with advanced disease in hospitals, the community and in residential and nursing homes (Bycroft and Brown, 1996, p. 434).

Euthanasia

The subject of euthanasia used to be divided into different categories: active and passive, voluntary and involuntary. Today what is considered as euthanasia is 'the intentional taking of life by a person other than the one requesting it' (Visser, 1995). When a person asks to have his or her life ended, this tends to be referred to as assisted suicide. By creating this second category, the problem has not become easier, but the distinctions are clearer.

In a survey of its readers conducted by the *Nursing Times*, 69 per cent of respondents said that patients in their area of work had requested euthanasia. When asked whether such requests were made to nursing or medical staff or to both groups, 59 per cent said to nursing staff, 5 per cent to medical staff, and 33 per cent to both medical and nursing staff. Some comments made by respondents 'expressed their feelings on the subject, often out of deeply felt and painful personal experiences which illustrated how the terminal illness and death of a loved one can change a person's detached professional view of [the subject]' (Pyne, 1995, p. 36).

This point was also emphasized by Finlay (1995), who maintained that at different times in their illness, patients have different and changing needs: 'the views of the medically well alter when they are medically ill'. For this reason, Finlay believes, 'professionals need a clear ethical framework around which to base their communication with patients over treatment options and approaches to care'. The ethical framework should be 'based on evaluation of risks and burdens against benefits' and 'can be used in all clinical practice to ensure that patients are respected as individuals'.

The debate in the UK centres round the question of whether euthanasia should be legalized. This debate was brought sharply into focus after the previously mentioned Tony Bland case. The House of Lords Select Committee on Medical Ethics (1994) made various recommendations following its permission for fluids and food to be withdrawn. Among them was that the interests of the individual cannot be separated from the interests of society as a whole and that individual cases are not sufficient reason to weaken the prohibition on intentional killing which protects us all.

Castledine (1994, p. 360) highlights more of the conclusions drawn by the House of Lords report which have implications for nursing:

- Palliative care services should be developed more widely, in particular in the community
- Decision-making should be a collective act, and nurses should be more actively taking part in this process
- Definitions such as persistent vegetative state should be more clearly defined and a code of practice should be available for the treatments of patients in this condition
- Decisions concerning the limiting of treatment should not be determined by considerations of resource availability. 'This factor will be warmly, if not a little cynically, accepted by nurses in management and practice areas' adds Castledine somewhat wryly
- Research into pain relief and symptom control should be encouraged

- Nurses who take on ethical responsibilities and who make ethical decisions should receive adequate education and training
- In order to maintain the dignity and self-respect of patients in long-term care, nurses should develop core standards for their care.

Good palliative care is essential for patients of any age and in any setting. Even though large numbers of nurses have enough training and skills for this care, their medical counterparts are often not similarly trained and skilled and this can lead to misunderstandings and friction (Anon, 1992). Only a very small proportion of dying patients have access to, or want to die in, hospices. It is therefore not surprising that many patients fear a lingering or painful death and ask to be allowed to die before they become too dependent or too distraught. Some would argue that this is a plea for help or for attention. Finlay (1995), says that 'the duty to care is the duty to listen'. 'No-one is obliged to request euthanasia; on the other hand, no-one should be denied the freedom to do so' (Pyne, 1995, p. 36). But are nurses well enough trained to hear the distinction between a plea for help and a genuine request to end life? Perhaps this is the real challenge for nurses.

The care of patients in PVS can be particularly distressing especially as it is not entirely clear what PVS is. Although distinctions have been drawn between PVS and a 'locked-in' state, the urgency of the recommendation made by the House of Lords, for a clear definition of the condition, is readily apparent.

While the case of Tony Bland progressed through the various legal stages, much was written about his situation. His parents had requested that he be allowed to die and his father had apparently asked, 'they say that where there's life there's hope – but where there's no hope, should there be life?' (Ellis, 1992, p. 42). Ellis suggested that in cases such as Tony Bland's, three questions should be asked and answered. 'What are the consequences of allowing this person to die, for himself or herself, for the immediate family, and for society?' 'Is allowing this person to die an acceptable (good) action?' 'What are the duties of the health care professionals to this person, the family, the professions, and to society?'

The concept of 'best interest' is often used to come to a decision, but on closer inspection Rose (1995, p. 149) suggests that this notion is far from clear. Establishing who are the 'experts' in any particular situation, as well as defining the 'incompetence' of the patient, are difficult tasks. Rose (1995, p. 149) also points out that the term 'best interest' is not used in relation 'to actual outcomes but rather in relation to the intended outcome of long-term good'. In this sense, Ellis' (1992, p. 41) questions are more complex than they appear at first sight. Issues such as a 'right to die', 'what is the meaning of life', and 'who can make decisions in controversial situations', need much more attention and debate. The contribution by nurses and nursing to the debates are crucial at every level, particularly as nurses are taking their role of advocates more seriously (Love, 1995).

One way of minimizing the dilemmas at the end of life is by having and using advance directives, or living wills. Such documents are not law in the UK, although in the USA, Canada, Australia and the Netherlands 'laws have been passed concerning the use of advance directives and health-care proxies' (Schlyter, 1992). The House of Lords Select Committee (1994) has also recommended that living wills should be taken into account when caring for people who have written such documents but who are no longer in a position to speak for themselves.

A living will gives a person increased self-control during a time when they may experience loss of control (Watt, 1995) and when 'quality of life is of more central concern, particularly if it is viewed in terms of its relationship to health and... life satisfaction, happiness and wellbeing' (Fox, 1994, p. 203). Bassett (1993) argues that over the last 200 years too much responsibility has been taken away from patients concerning the living and dying, and living wills are one way of returning this responsibility to them.

Resuscitation

Stories abound in the nursing and medical literature of patients who, either implicitly or explicitly, had stated that they would like to die but when they arrested, were resuscitated (Schultz, 1997). The question usually posed then is, 'why'?

According to Schultz (1997), a survey conducted in Sweden in 1990 in all 92 acute care hospitals, found 191 different symbols and 31 written code words to indicate the not for resuscitation (NFR) status of patients.

Cardiopulmonary resuscitation (CPR) has become possible because of technology, but for many people, CPR is not an appropriate intervention. When faced with 'the problem of determining under what conditions, according to what criteria and by whom' (Schultz, 1997, p. 231) such decisions are made, the outcome is one of confusion rather than clarity.

A statement issued jointly by the Royal College of Nursing (RCN) and the British Medical Association (BMA) in 1993 (RCN, 1993a), the following guidelines are advocated:

> It is appropriate to consider a do-not-resuscitate (DNR) decision in the following circumstances:
>
> a) where the patient's condition indicates that effective cardiopulmonary resuscitation (CPR) is unlikely to be successful
> b) where CPR is not in accord with the recorded, sustained wishes of the patient who is mentally competent
> c) where successful CPR is likely to be followed by a length and quality of life which would not be acceptable to the patient.

Schutz (1994) believes that the practice of not involving patients in resuscitation decisions has usually been defended on the grounds that 'such involvement may be harmful for patients as it may spoil their enjoyment of their last few weeks of life' (p. 1075). She goes on to quote Loewy (1991), who states that 'involving patients in resuscitation decisions may be more painful for health care professionals than for patients' (Schutz, 1994, p. 1078).

The problem of CPR is a typical end of life problem which technology and science, rather than medicine, have created. The procedure is not in question in emergency situations: it is applied anyway. But in the long-term and chronically ill (Kent, 1996), the sick elderly and the severely ill, a decision of NFR is much more difficult to make and is more controversial.

The RCN/BMA (RCN, 1993a) statement says that 'DNR orders may be a potent source of misunderstanding and dissent among doctors, nurses and others involved in the care of patients'. Schutz (1994, p. 1078) says that this is 'usually the result of a failure to address the issue at the right time'. Tackling this problem needs all the tact and communication skills available but, above all, a team approach is vital if patients, their families and those close to them are to feel confident and trust is to be maintained by all involved.

Organ transplantation

In the league of scarce resources, organ transplants are classed as the paradigmatic case (Dickenson, 1994, p. 207). For lay people it is easy to see that organ transplant decisions have to be made entirely on medical grounds, but as Dickenson (1994, p. 208) shows, this is far from the case: in 1986 in the USA, 'Baby Jesse' was refused a heart transplant on the grounds that 'his parents were unmarried teenagers with a criminal history and drug abuse problem. They were judged incapable of providing the necessary follow-up procedures, such as punctual administration of immuno-suppressive medications.' The case of Laura Davies mentioned above brought the debate about organ donation to the fore in the UK.

Organ transplantation can be offered to patients for the wrong reasons, for instance 'as a way of keeping hope alive and denying mortality' (Iliffe and Swan, 1993, p. 60). Iliffe and Swan (1993) list this as one of the special considerations which apply to organ donation. Others include the following requirements: that patients should be allowed to refuse assessment for transplant without recrimination; that they know what is in their best interest so as to give informed consent; that helping patients to maintain a positive attitude in the waiting period can conflict with the ethical requirement to discuss the risks of rejection and death with them; and that patients often seem to need to make an impression of being good and worthy of the transplant.

In their very thoughtful chapter, Iliffe and Swan (1993) discuss several of the more intangible aspects of organ transplantation. Among other things, they say that, 'the considerable financial resources put into the transplant programme finally benefit a relatively small number of people, and no human audit is taken of those who were not eligible for assessment, those who failed to meet the assessment criteria, those who died while waiting and those for whom transplant was unsuccessful' (p. 69). The ethical questions revolve around these issues. The high cost of transplants compared to other, simpler measures of enhancing the quality of life for many more people, is a point which always needs to be kept in mind.

Turner (1993) reinforces the claim which Iliffe and Swan (1993, p. 61) also make, that patients and relatives need more information about the possible complications following the transplant. It may be that patients and families have been given as much information as possible, but that under the circumstances, they simply could not absorb this information for various practical and psychological reasons.

In the case of Laura Davies, Turner (1993) quotes Baroness Warnock as saying 'that it would be dishonest to pretend that such a multiple transplant [the second, six-organ transplant carried out in the USA] could have been considered anything other than experimental' (p. 18). Questions about the purpose of treatment and of the quality of life and respect for the person, need to be addressed again and again. Turner (1993, p. 18) asks, 'could nurses help to safeguard the rights of the children within this very sensitive area of organ transplantation?' Nurses at Great Ormond Street Children's Hospital in London have learned that 'it is both wise and possible to bring children, even as young as three, into the decision-making process' (p. 18). What is possible with children must be possible with adults. It may be argued that the language may need to be as simple with adults as it is with children, because when faced with such decisions, we are all 'children'.

For transplants to be possible, the less glamorous aspect of 'organ retrieval' is necessary and this topic attracts periodic discussion among nurses. The criteria for brain death are laid down in law (RCN, 1993b), but ethical issues arise because of the speed with which it is necessary to act. Durman and Hudson (1993) describe the guidelines developed at the Royal Devon and Exeter Hospital. These give clear instructions for every part of the organ retrieval process when a potential donor is admitted to the hospital.

In Britain, there is a 'chronic and worsening shortfall of donor kidneys' (Evans, 1993, p. 34). Quite why this is happening is not clear. The editor of the *Bulletin of Medical Ethics* (1994a, p. 1) stated that 'organ donation in Germany dropped 20% this spring when Protestant bishops suggested that brain death was an invention of doctors for their own purposes and did not really represent death'. He suggested that organ donation is not in keeping with the respect we owe the dead. In an ethics course for qualified undergraduate nurses studying for various nursing degrees, the question as to whether or not they would be prepared to be donors if the circumstances were there, was asked. Two-thirds of the class said no. Asked if they would accept organ transplants if they needed them, they also said no. In the discussion which followed, the reasons they gave were that they preferred to maintain their bodily integrity. Perhaps this is an indication of the direction in which people who either think about the issues or are aware of the consequences of transplants may be heading.

End of life issues in the Netherlands

It is feasible to assume that for most nurses in the Netherlands many of the problems discussed so far are very familiar, with the one exception of euthanasia. The Netherlands are always quoted as an example of how euthanasia is either helpful, 'euthanasia as practised in the Netherlands is caring at its very best' (Pyne, 1995, p. 38), or that 'there is disturbing evidence not only of a high incidence of euthanasia in Holland but also of widespread breach of the guidelines' (Gormally, 1994, p. 161). The practice of euthanasia in the Netherlands, therefore, colours the discussion of all the end of life issues.

The guidelines which govern physicians in the practice of euthanasia in the Netherlands were published in 1984 by the Royal Dutch Medical Association (KNMG). The five points considered to be conditions in which euthanasia (meaning 'voluntary euthanasia') accorded with medical ethics are:

1. The request must be made of the patient's free will, and not result from pressure by others.

2. The request must be 'well-considered', and not be based on a misunderstanding of diagnosis or prognosis.
3. The request must be 'durable', and not arise from impulse or temporary depression.
4. The patient must be experiencing 'unacceptable suffering'; he must feel the suffering to be 'persistent, unbearable and hopeless'.
5. The doctor must consult with a colleague before performing euthanasia, and report it to the legal authorities afterwards as a non-natural death (Keown, 1992, pp. 160–1).

In 1991 the government commissioned a survey of the practice of euthanasia, chaired by Attorney-General Remmelink, which published its report in 1992. The results of that survey are widely used as the basis for discussion of the practice of euthanasia in the Netherlands.

> The Survey shows that for the calendar year 1990, there were 2,300 cases of (voluntary) euthanasia and 400 cases of assisted suicide. There were... over 8,000 cases in which doctors administered morphine, and almost 8,000 cases in which they withheld or withdrew treatment 'explicitly' or 'partly' with the intent to shorten life. ...The Survey revealed over 1,000 cases in which doctors stated that they had terminated life without the explicit request of the patient (van der Maas *et al.*, 1992, p. 1).

These figures should be seen in perspective. The Netherlands have a population of approximately 14 million people. In 1990, 42 per cent of deaths took place at home, 41 per cent in hospital and the remainder in nursing homes (*Bulletin of Medical Ethics*, 1994b). Nursing homes are often seen to be the place for palliative care and care of the dying. Statistics from the Ministry of Public Health, Welfare and Sports (Rijswijk, 1996) show that between 1988 and 1996 the number of beds in nursing homes has barely changed, but the number of personnel employed in them has increased from 79,000 to 96,000.

According to Sheldon (1995), a member of the largest nursing organization in the Netherlands, Nieuwe Unie '91 (Nu91), is quoted as saying that 'euthanasia is often misunderstood in foreign countries. Euthanasia is not easy in the Netherlands – it is very complicated' (p. 16). Nurses are frequently confronted with requests for euthanasia (Sheldon, 1993) and they have to respond. In order to help nurses, Nu91 (1993) has published guidelines for nurses (in conjunction with the KNMG). This document mentions that nurses' 'continuing involvement' and 'special knowledge' are 'highly desirable' when they have to consider a request for euthanasia. 'If a nurse disagrees with a doctor's refusal to perform euthanasia, it advises the nurse to seek a second opinion from another doctor, ward sister or hospital director to avoid a psychological conflict of duties from which there is no exit' (Sheldon, 1993, p. 15).

The guidelines 'make it clear that while both the decision to proceed with euthanasia and its implementation lies with the doctor, the nurse who gives continuing care for the patient should preferably be involved' (Sheldon, 1993, p. 15). Indeed, in the test case against Dr Henk Prins (Sheldon, 1994), he made it clear that the nurses who cared for the baby he killed played an important role in his decision.

Several cases of euthanasia in the Netherlands have become well known because they have been widely disseminated. Dr Prins had followed the guidelines strictly, consulting with several colleagues on the chances of survival of a four-day-old baby who had several disabilities including spina bifida, hydro-cephalus and brain damage. Dr Prins could have prescribed increasing doses of morphine, but he argued that this would only have prolonged her pain and suffering and created increasing uncertainty about the moment of death. Giving her one injection meant that she died in the arms of her mother. In this way Dr Prins made himself culpable before the law (Sheldon, 1994).

In March 1995 BBC television showed the documentary *Death on Request*, which was a record of the last months of Cees van Wendel de Joode, showing his death by injection, given by his GP Dr Wilfred van Oijen (Sheldon, 1995).

While these cases clearly argue for euthanasia, some people in the Netherlands are not convinced in the same way. At the conference, 'Euthanasia: Towards a European Consensus?' in November 1995 in Brussels, some Dutch speakers commented that the Dutch experience is not easily transferable to other coun-tries not in sympathy with the guidelines in the Netherlands; that good palliative care can never be a substitute for euthanasia;

that once euthanasia has been officially sanctioned, it develops
an impetus of its own; that conflicts of duties are becoming
clear: the duty to preserve life versus the duty to kill – obeying
the law versus respecting the patient; that in cases which were
not reported, colleagues were consulted less; and that the incidence of palliative care in the Netherlands has dramatically
increased in recent years. The large increase in personnel in
nursing homes in recent years must bear on this topic.

A recurring question at the conference concerned the knowledge base for end of life decisions. Perhaps the practice of
euthanasia in the Netherlands is pushing in the direction of
better practice generally, showing, as is so often the case, that
ethics follows practice and does not lead it.

End of life issues in Switzerland

The Swiss Nurses Association (SBK – ASI) published its code
of practice in 1990. Apart from the actual code, the document
also contains short explanations of ethical principles, recommended reading, the ICN *Code for Nurses* and the UN Declaration of Human Rights, 1948.

Switzerland has a population of just over 7 million people
and belongs neither to the European Union nor the United
Nations; the latter is for reasons of housing the headquarters
of the UN, the former because a majority voted against entry
in recent referenda.

The Swiss health care system is organized at cantonal level,
with 26 cantons, each featuring different systems. Although a
new federal health insurance law implemented in 1996 demanded, for the first time, compulsory health insurance for all, its
interpretation by the different cantons varies considerably.

As yet, in the majority of cantons nurses are either not
mentioned at all as health care professionals or they figure as
assistants to physicians. In the realm of nursing education there
are plans to offer university level programmes within the next
five years and the first of these to be offered at Basle university received approval in 1997. It is therefore not surprising
that nurses have had little impact on public or medical
decision-making in health care issues.

Care of the dying

The health care system in Switzerland relies on obligatory health insurance for everyone.

Although palliative care has long existed in Switzerland, it was not until 1988 that the Schweizerische Gesellschaft für Palliative Medizin (Swiss Association for Palliative Medicine) came into being (Serena, 1989). The aims of the association are to: develop palliative care without making it a speciality; train and educate medical and nursing personnel; exchange information; develop the methods of care; and inform health care personnel as well as the general public. In 1993 the first home care centre for the care of the dying was started in Sion (canton Valais) (Kocher, 1994). This centre employs 15 people and domiciliary care is offered by a team of specialists. It acts as a centre for information and documentation, offers psychological and social help and serves as a research and training resource (Kocher, 1994).

As a subject, care of the dying is frequently discussed in nursing journals, the literature and in seminars (Jost, 1995).

Euthanasia

The word used to describe euthanasia is *Sterbehilfe*, meaning 'helping to die'.

The Schweizerische Akademie der Medizinischen Wissenschaften (SAMW: Swiss Academy of Medical Sciences) has guidelines for the care of dying and cerebrally damaged patients (SAZ, 1995). These guidelines were first published in 1976 and revised in 1981, 1988 and 1993. The 1995 text is significant in several areas. Compared with the earlier guidelines, the 1995 text asks physicians not to prolong life for those who are dying, whereas before, this was only considered a possibility. Living wills (*Patiententestament*) must now be respected, whereas before they need not have been. Assisted suicide is definitely excluded and physicians should consult with relatives and the caring team regarding any decisions which may be irreversible. Thus the duties of physicians have been more clearly defined and according to Ernst (1996), their freedom has been curbed, but the responsibility for making the final decisions is now shared and no longer rests on the physician alone.

A Member of Parliament, Victor Ruffy, tabled a motion in September 1994 which would regulate assisted suicide. The government may have to debate and rule further on the question of euthanasia.

A question which disturbs nurses is what to do when a dying patient refuses their care, such as being turned (Spichiger, 1995). Spichiger suggests in her study that nurses tended to show an unthinking and paternalistic attitude. More discussion on the subject of the care of the dying and sharing of experiences through, for example, reflective practice, would be one way of helping to make the patients' dying easier. Remmers (1996) also suggests that an ethic of care needs to be established in nursing so that 'helping to die' is not a major problem for nurses.

Organ transplants

Switzerland has six centres where organ transplants are carried out. In 1996 a total of 357 organs were transplanted and more than half of them were kidneys. But in January 1997, 464 people were on waiting lists. Schlumpf (1997) believes that transplants suffer because people do not want to face illness and death. Swisstransplant, the organization responsible for co-ordinating the transplant programme, believes that an advertising campaign will help. The SAMW published two documents in 1996 concerning transplants and a new law should be introduced in the future which should help to remedy the situation. In the documents the role of nurses is not mentioned (personal communication), but it is clearly a part of patient care about which they are concerned (Haupt, 1994; Gonseth, 1996).

Conclusion

End of life problems have always existed, but modern medicine has made them much more difficult. Death has become the Big Problem. We no longer believe in a better life hereafter to look forward to, therefore all our efforts are concentrated on this life.

At present, our efforts to make the last stages of life dignified still have a cloak of morality about them, but in all of the problematic cases which reach the media, a financial aspect is always involved. In a market-led society people do inevitably have a price tag and establishing how much someone is worth is really what we are saying in relation to the various techniques described in this chapter. The individual is seen and treated as an isolated entity to the detriment of society at large.

Perhaps the real moral and ethical challenges for nurses, and health care workers generally, is how to maintain the dignity of, and respect for, the individual person, who is also a member of, and has responsibilities to, a family, a community and a society, each of whom rightly claim the person as their own.

Although political and economic issues play some part, many of the problems involving end of life issues arise because of poor communication. Essentially, this means that we are no longer competent to talk with and listen to each other. By fostering these aspects, nurses will make a much bigger impact on end of life decisions than may yet be envisaged. This takes empathy, compassion and courage.

Acknowledgements

I would like to thank Dr Arie van der Arend, Dr Annemarie Kesselring and Maya Shaha for their help with comments and documents in the preparation of this chapter.

References

Anonymous (1992) 'A matter of life and death' ('Open Door' column), *Nursing Times*, **88**(27): 55.

Bassett, C.C. (1993) 'The living will: implications for nurses', *British Journal of Nursing*, **2**(13): 688–91.

Bulletin of Medical Ethics (1994a) 'Editorial', **98**:1.

Bulletin of Medical Ethics (1994b) 'Ending life in Holland', **103**: 5.

Bycroft, L. and Brown, J.G. (1996) 'Care of the dying', in Tschudin, V. (ed.) *Nursing the Patient with Cancer*, 2nd edn. (Prentice Hall: Hemel Hempstead), pp. 419–37.

Callahan, D. (1990) *What Kind of Life? The Limits of Medical Progress*. (Simon & Schuster: New York).

Castledine, G. (1994) 'House of Lords' response to end-of-life issues', *British Journal of Nursing*, **3**(7): 359–60.

Dickenson, D. (1994) Nurse time as a scarce health care resource, in Hunt, G. (ed.) *Ethical Issues in Nursing*. (Routledge: London), pp. 207–17.

Durman, R. and Hudson, S. (1993) 'Protocol for loss', *Nursing Times*, **89**(45): 50–2.

Ellis, P. (1992) 'Living a dilemma', *Nursing Standard*, **7**(12): 41–3.

Ernst, C. (1996) 'Eingrenzung der Entscheidungsfreiheit, aber auch Entlastung der Alleinverantwortung', *VSAO Bulletin ASMAC*, **5**: 5–6.

Evans, M. (1993) 'Moral costs', *Nursing Times*, **89**(37): 34–5.

Finlay, I. (1995) 'Autonomy and the duty to care: a practical perspective', Paper given at Euthanasia: Towards a European Consensus? Conference, 24–5 November, Hotel Astoria, Brussels.

Fox, J. (1994) 'Professional acceptance of living wills to be encouraged', *British Journal of Nursing*, **3**(5): 202–3.

Gill, S. (1994) 'Are we obliged to keep very premature infants alive?', *British Journal of Midwifery*, **2**(9): 448–52.

Gonseth, R. (1996) 'Ein unhaltbarer Zustand!', *Soziale Medizin SM*, **23**(1): 5, 33.

Gormally, L. (ed.) (1994) *Euthanasia, Clinical Practice and the Law*. (The Linacre Centre for Health Care Ethics: London).

Grimley, I. (1995) 'Dilemmas of care', *Nursing Times*, **91**(18): 42–3.

Haupt, J.C. (1994) 'Hirntod – Organspende', *Pflegezeitschrift*, **47**(7): 401–4.

Hospice Information Service (1997) *Directory of Hospice Services in the UK and Republic of Ireland*. (St Christopher's Hospice: London).

House of Lords (1994) 'Report of the Select Committee on Medical Ethics', 1(237) (HMSO: London).

Hunt, J. (1993) 'Quality of the patient's life versus the quest for a cure', *British Journal of Nursing*, **2**(16): 819–22.

Iliffe, J. and Swan, P. (1993) 'Heart and heart–lung transplantation', in Tschudin, V. (ed.) *Ethics: Aspects of Nursing Care*. (Scutari Press: London), pp. 56–71.

Jost, W. (1995) 'Palliative Pflege im Spannungsfeld zwischen Pflegeteam Arzt und Angehörigen', *Nova*, **11**: 12–15.

Kent, M.A. (1996) 'The ethical arguments concerning the artificial ventilation of patients with motor neurone disease', *Nursing Ethics*, **3**(4): 317–28.

Keown, J. (1992) 'The law and practice of euthanasia in the Netherlands', *Law Quarterly Review*, **108**: 51–78, cited in Gormally, L.

(ed.) (1994) *Euthanasia, Clinical Practice and the Law.* (The Linacre Centre: London).

Kocher, B. (1994) 'Approcher la mort avec sérénité', *Krankenpflege/ Soins Infirmiers*, **11**: 62–4.

Loewy, E.H. (1991) 'Involving patients in do not resuscitate (DNR) decisions: an old issue raising its ugly head', *Journal of Medical Ethics*, **17**: 156–60.

Love, M.B. (1995) 'Patient advocacy at the end of life', *Nursing Ethics*, **2**(1): 3–9.

van der Maas, P.J. *et al.* (1992) 'Euthanasia and other medical decisions at the end of life', *Health Policy*, **22**: 1–2, cited in Gormally, L. (ed.) (1994) *Euthanasia, Clinical Practice and the Law.* (The Linacre Centre: London).

Nu91 (1993) *Euthanasie-richtlijnen; Arts-verpleegkundige.* (Nieuwe Unie: Utrecht).

Paintin, D. (1991) 'The implications of the new legislation on abortion', *Maternal and Child Health*, **16**(7): 221–4.

Pyne, R. (1995) 'The euthanasia debate: how NT readers view the issues', *Nursing Times*, **91**(35): 36–8.

RCN (1993a) *Cardiopulmonary Resuscitation: A Statement from the RCN and the BMA.* (RCN/BMA: London).

RCN (1993b) 'Harvesting of organs: a review of the legal, ethical and nursing issues', *Issues in Nursing and Health*, **19** (Royal College of Nursing: London).

Remmers, H. (1996) 'Sterbehilfe – ethische Herausforderungen an pflegerisches Handeln und institutionelle Rahmenbedingungen', *Pflege*, **9**(4): 267–77.

Rijswijk (1996) *Zorg in getal 1996*, Ministry of Public Health, Welfare and Sports, May.

Rose, P. (1995) 'Best interests: a concept analysis and its implications for ethical decision-making in nursing', *Nursing Ethics*, **2**(2): 149–60.

SAMW (1995) 'Medizinisch-ethische Richtlinien für die Organtransplantationen', *Schweizerische Aerztezeitung*, **96**(35): 1389–91.

SAZ (1995) 'Medizinisch-ethische Richtlinien für die ärztliche Betreuung sterbender und zerebral schwerst geschädigter Patienten', *Schweizerische Aerztezeitung*, **76**(29/30): 1223–5.

Schlumpf, R. (1997) 'Weiterhin Mangel an Transplantationsorganen', *Neue Zürcher Zeitung*, 7 February, 13.

Schlyter, C. (1992) *Advance Directives and AIDS: Centre for Medical Law and Ethics.* (King's College: London).

Schultz, L. (1997) 'Not for resuscitation: two decades of challenge for nursing ethics and practice', *Nursing Ethics*, **4**(3): 227–38.

Schutz, S.E. (1994) 'Patient involvement in resuscitation decisions', *British Journal of Nursing*, **3**(20): 1075–9.

Serena, P. (1989) 'Pflege, die nur noch lindern will', *Krankenpflege/ Soins Infirmiers*, **11**: 10–13.
Shamash, J. (1995) 'Measures for comfort and joy', *Nursing Times*, **91**(33): 14–15.
Sheldon, T. (1993) 'Last rights', *Nursing Times*, **89**(44): 14–15.
Sheldon, T. (1994) 'Final reckoning', *Nursing Times*, **90**(35): 20.
Sheldon, T. (1995) 'A peaceful, public death', *Nursing Times*, **91**(11): 16.
Spichiger, E. (1995) 'Sterbende pflegen... und wenn sie nein sagen?', *Pflege*, **8**(3): 203–12.
Thiroux, J. (1995) *Ethics: Theory and Practice*, 5th edn. (Prentice Hall: Englewood Cliffs, N.J.).
Turner, T. (1993) 'Laura's legacy', *Nursing Times*, **89**(47): 18.
Visser, J. (1995) 'The termination of life by a doctor in the Netherlands', Paper given at Euthanasia: Towards a European Consensus? Conference, 24–5 November, Hotel Astoria, Brussels.
Watt, P. (1995) 'Living wills: how do they inform care?', *British Journal of Nursing*, **4**(19): 1156–9.

Suggestions for further reading

Age Concern (1988) *The Living Will: Consent to Treatment at the End of Life*. (Edward Arnold: London).
Fuchs, V.R. (1974 and 1983) *Who Shall Live? Health, Economics, and Social Choice*. (Basic Books: New York).
Gormally, L. (ed.) (1994) *Euthanasia, Clinical Practice and the Law*. (The Linacre Centre: London).
de Hennezel, M. (1995) *La Mort Intime*. (Robert Laffont: Paris).
Rachels, J. (1986) *The End of Life; Euthanasia and Morality*. (Oxford University Press: Oxford).
Schwartzenberg, L. (1994) *Face à la Détresse*. (Fayard: Paris).

Appendix

Extract from *The Midwives Code of Practice* (UKCC, 1994, pp. 4–6) incorporating the Activities etc.

The activities of a midwife are defined in the European Midwives Directive 80/155/EEC Article 4:

Member states shall ensure that midwives are at least entitled to take up and pursue the following activities:

5.1 to provide sound family planning information and advice;

5.2 to diagnose pregnancies and monitor normal pregnancies; to carry out examinations necessary for the monitoring of the development of normal pregnancies;

5.3 to prescribe or advise on the examinations necessary for the earliest possible diagnosis of pregnancies at risk;

5.4 to provide a programme of parenthood preparation and a complete preparation for childbirth including advice on hygiene and nutrition;

5.5 to care for and assist the mother during labour and to monitor the condition of the fetus in utero by the appropriate clinical and technical means;

5.6 to conduct spontaneous deliveries including where required an episiotomy and in urgent cases a breech delivery;

5.7 to recognise the warning signs of abnormality in the mother or infant which necessitate referral to a doctor and to assist the latter where appropriate; to take the necessary emergency measures in the doctor's absence, in particular the manual removal of the placenta, possibly followed by manual examination of the uterus;

5.8 to examine and care for the new-born infant; to take all initiatives which are necessary in case of need and to carry out where necessary immediate resuscitation;

5.9 to care for and monitor the progress of the mother in the postnatal period and to give all necessary advice to the mother on infant care to enable her to ensure the optimum progress of the new-born infant;

5.10 to carry out the treatment prescribed by a doctor;

5.11 to maintain all necessary records.

Index